Nursing in the
Community

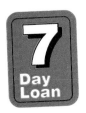

7
Day
Loan

Nursing in the Community

An essential guide to practice

Edited by

Sue Chilton BNurs, RN, DN, HV, MSc, PGCE, DNT
Senior Lecturer, University of Central England in Birmingham and
Staff Nurse, District Nursing Service, Cotswold
and Vale Primary Care Trust, UK

Karen Melling MA, PGCEA, RDNT, PWT, DN, RN
Senior Lecturer, University of Gloucestershire, Cheltenham, UK

Dee Drew RN, DN, MSc
Senior Lecturer, University of Wolverhampton, Wolverhampton, UK

Ann Clarridge MSc, BSc (Hons), PGCEA, DNT, RN, DN
Principal Lecturer, London South Bank University, London, UK

A member of the Hodder Headline Group

LONDON

First published in Great Britain in 2004 by
Arnold, a member of the Hodder Headline Group,
338 Euston Road, London NW1 3BH

http://www.arnoldpublishers.com

Distributed in the United States of America by
Oxford University Press Inc.,
198 Madison Avenue, New York, NY10016
Oxford is a registered trademark of Oxford University Press

Whilst the advice and information in this book are believed to be true and
accurate at the date of going to press, neither the authors nor the publisher
can accept any legal responsibility or liability for any errors or omissions
that may be made. In particular (but without limiting the generality of the
preceding disclaimer) every effort has been made to check drug dosages;
however, it is still possible that errors have been missed. Furthermore,
dosage schedules are constantly being revised and new side-effects
recognized. For these reasons the reader is strongly urged to consult the
drug companies' printed instructions before administering any of the drugs
recommended in this book.

British Library Cataloguing in Publication Data
A catalogue record for this book is available from the British Library

Library of Congress Cataloging-in-Publication Data
A catalog record for this book is available from the Library of Congress

ISBN 0 340 81043 2

1 2 3 4 5 6 7 8 9 10

Commissioning Editor: Georgina Bentliff
Development Editor: Heather Smith
Project Editor: Wendy Rooke
Production Controller: Lindsay Smith
Cover Design: Amina Dudhia

Typeset in 9.5/12pt Berling by Phoenix Photosetting, Chatham, Kent
Printed and bound in Spain

What do you think about this book? Or any other Arnold title?
Please send your comments to feedback.arnold@hodder.co.uk

Contents

Chapter 1

Setting the scene: an introduction   1
Dee Drew, Sue Chilton, Ann Clarridge and Karen Melling
Social and political influences – demographic influences – community specialist practice

Chapter 2

New ways of working   7
Anne Smith
Changes in service delivery – organisational culture – leadership – managing change

Chapter 3

Nursing in a community environment   17
Sue Chilton
Factors influencing community nursing – health needs assessment – responding to local needs – roles of specialist community nurses – ensuring quality of care

Chapter 4

Personal safety in the community   29
Dee Drew
Preparation for home visits – personal safety – non-confrontational behaviour – manual handling – reporting of incidents

Chapter 5

Therapeutic relationships   41
Patricia Wilson and Sue Miller
The features of therapeutic relationships – maintaining boundaries – promoting a positive experience – the nature of care – the impact of policy changes

Chapter 6

Working collaboratively   53
Ann Clarridge and Elaine Ryder
Relevant government policy – defining collaboration – the interface of collaborative care – collaborative skills and attitudes

Contributors

Sandra Baulcomb RN, RM, DN Cert, PWT Cert, Cert Ed, RDN Tutor, BA (Hons), MSc
Lecturer, University of Hull, Hull, UK

Sandra Burley BA (Hons), RN, RM, DN, RNT
Lecturer, University of Hull, Hull, UK

Sue Chilton BNurs, RN, DN, HV, MSc, PGCE, DNT
Senior Lecturer, University of Central England in Birmingham and Staff Nurse, District Nursing Service, Cotswold and Vale Primary Care Trust, UK

Ann Clarridge MSc, BSc (Hons), PGCEA, DNT, RN, DN
Principal Lecturer, South Bank University, London, UK

Dee Drew RN, DN, MSc
Senior Lecturer, University of Wolverhampton, Wolverhampton, UK

Judy Gleeson MA, BSc (Hons), PG Dip Nursing (Education), RHV, RN
Senior Lecturer, University of Gloucestershire, Cheltenham, UK

Karen Hunter BA (Hons), RHV, RN
Clinical Governance Coordinator, South Warwickshire Primary Care Trust, Warwickshire, UK

Karen Melling MA, PGCEA, RDNT, PWT, DN, RN
Senior Lecturer, University of Gloucestershire, Cheltenham, UK

Sue Miller RN, RSCN, Dip Nursing, DNCert, Cert Ed, BSc (Hons) Nursing Studies, MSc Child Health Nursing
Senior Lecturer, University of Hertfordshire, Hatfield, UK

Jenny Parry MSc, RN, RM, NDN, PWT, DNT, NP
Principal Lecturer, Canterbury Christ Church University College, Canterbury, UK

Judith Parsons MSc, BA, RN, DNT, DNCert, PWT, NP
Senior Lecturer, Canterbury Christ Church University College, Canterbury, UK

Susan Rouse BSc (Hons), RN, RHV, Postgrad Dip Child Protection HETC
Lecturer, University of Hull, Hull, UK

Elaine Ryder RN, NCDN, CPT, Cert Ed, RNT, DNT, BA, MSc, ILT
Principal Lecturer, Oxford Brookes University, Oxford, UK

Anne Smith BSc (Hons) (Dist. Nurse) PGCE, RN
Lecturer in Primary Care, University of Reading, Reading, UK

Milly Smith MSc, Cert Ed, SRN, QIDN, CPT
Principal Lecturer, School of Health, University of Wolverhampton, Wolverhampton, UK

Patricia Wilson RN, NDN, PWT, BEd (Hons) Nursing Education, MSc
Senior Lecturer, University of Hertfordshire, Hatfield, UK

Foreword

Nurses working in all community settings are experiencing unprecedented change. It is driven by many factors: demographic shifts, higher rates of chronic disease, health policy, increasingly better engaged patients, social and economic developments, and progress in medical and other technologies and in nursing practice – to name the key factors. The interplay of these variables is dynamic and inter-dependent. Health policy, for example, addresses the impact of changes in the demographic make-up both in the population and in the workforce, while changing social mores and expectations demand health policies that recognise the primacy of the patient at the heart of decision making and choice. For nurses, each of the factors is powerful enough in its own right to prompt significant change: together, they form an irresistible force. The demand for nurses and expectations of nursing will rise exponentially as the new world unfolds. More nurses will be working outside of hospitals; more of them will have specialist or expert skills; many will continue as generalists offering flexible and accessible care in a variety of settings including the home. Nurses will practice in multi-disciplinary teams as members and as leaders; their work will cross organisational boundaries, and will be built on partnerships – none more vital than the partnerships with their patients and the communities they serve. They will help patients understand the choices available to them, and in expanding their skills and expertise, they themselves will increase the options on offer. We shall see more nurse entrepreneurs offering family health services or primary care for vulnerable groups. We shall see nurses as care managers, overseeing all aspects of provision for at-risk older people.

This book provides a timely resource on the context and processes of working in the community for those new to this environment, and is an important reminder for those not so new. As is made clear, nursing outside of hospital isn't just a change of setting. It is a different way of thinking, of acting and of being with local people and communities so that capacity and resources for health are increased and enhanced.

Though we speak of future needs, let us not be daunted by how much there is to do. Let us instead be encouraged by how far we have come. This book reflects powerful developments in nursing practice in the community that have taken place in recent years. It shows that none are more likely to adapt to and adopt change than community nurses themselves, who understand more than most what will best improve the care of their patients.

Sarah Mullally 2004

Acknowledgements

The idea for this book originated from the many enquiries that members of the Association of District Nurse Educators (ADNE) received requesting further information on working and 'surviving' in the community. With this in mind, all the contributors hope that this guide to practice will prove useful.

The book could not have been written without the ongoing support of the members of the Association of District Nurse Educators (ADNE) www.adne.com and from experts representing the various disciplines from the community specialist pathways.

Note on terminology and abbreviations

Below is an explanation of some of the terms favoured in the text of this book.

Patient: It is recognised that some groups of community nurses use other terminology in preference to patient, such as client or user.

Community specialist nurses: This term is intended to include occupational health nurses, health visitors, public health nurses, community children's nurses, community learning disability nurses, community psychiatric nurses, school nurses, district nurses, and general practice nurses. These practitioners have undertaken further programmes of education, which have been registered or recorded with the Nursing and Midwifery Council.

Community staff nurses: These qualified nurses work in teams under the guidance of a community specialist nurse.

She: Nurses are referred to throughout as she, although it is recognised that there are many male community nurses working in Britain. The use of both he and she would have been clumsy, and to use 'he' by preference would have seemed inappropriate when most nurses are female.

The following sets of initials have been used in the text when making reference to literature published by these bodies: BMA: British Medical Association; CPHVA: Community Practitioners and Health Visitors Association; DHSS: Department of Health and Social Security; DOE: Department of Education; DOH: Department of Health; HMSO: Her Majesty's Stationery Office; HSE: Health and Safety Executive; HVA: Health Visitors Association; NHS: National Health Service; NHSME: NHS Management Executive; NMC Nursing and Midwifery Council; RCGP: Royal College of General Practitioners; RCN: Royal College of Nursing; UKCC: UK Central Council for Nursing, Midwifery and Health Visiting.

Setting the scene: an introduction

Dee Drew, Sue Chilton, Ann Clarridge and Karen Melling

These are exciting and challenging times for community nurses. *Liberating the Talents* (DOH 2002) provides a framework for the expansion of clinical roles and calls for greater freedom to encourage creativity. This book has been designed to support staff who may be new to working in a community setting and is an essential guide to practice. We envisage it will be useful for community staff nurses and nurses moving from an acute work environment to take up a community post. These 'front-line' nurses might be working in any of the following disciplines: occupational health nursing, health visiting, community children's nursing, community learning disability nursing, community psychiatric nursing, school nursing, district nursing and general practice nursing. Such nurses are not only responsible for personal care of patients and for a range of clinical interventions, but also for the assessment of health needs, planning, delivery and evaluation of direct care for individuals and groups of patients. In addition, they may be responsible for mentoring students, and directing and supervising the work of support workers.

The aim of the book is to develop and support a practitioner so she can function safely and effectively in a range of primary care/community settings. The authors take an inclusive approach, working from a health and social needs perspective and demonstrating the involvement of patients, professionals and non-professionals.

A range of topics relating to professional issues in community nursing is addressed. The text reflects recent and current government health and social care policy reforms and the effect of these on the roles and responsibilities of community nurses.

Community nursing is seen in the context of political, social and environmental influences. Interpersonal and practical skills, as well as the knowledge base required by community nurses, are critically analysed and linked to relevant theory. Examples and exercises relating to the range of community disciplines are included throughout the book to stimulate the reader's creative thinking.

Topics covered include new ways of working, nursing in a community environment, personal safety, therapeutic relationships, working collaboratively, conceptual approaches to care, professional issues in community nursing, public health and health promotion.

SOCIAL AND POLITICAL INFLUENCES UPON COMMUNITY NURSING

The economic crisis of the 1970s led to the first real major reforms in the National Health Service (NHS). The centralisation of administrative power led to dissatisfaction amongst NHS employees. In 1976 the Resource Allocation Working Party reviewed the allocation of funds and began the move away from the focus upon London hospitals. The then government advocated a change of balance in services, emphasizing the need to prioritise older people, people with learning disabilities and the mentally ill (DHSS 1977). The importance of strengthening service provision within the community was clearly stated. In 1979 Margaret Thatcher's Conservative government was elected to power. The Conservative election manifesto made no statement relating to health policy.

With underpinning values of efficiency savings and cost improvement, the NHS in the early 1980s was bureaucratic and seriously underfunded (Lawton *et al.* 2000). In 1982, Roy Griffiths, a successful manager but with limited experience of health care management, was charged with the review of the management of the NHS. It was widely thought by the government that poor management was behind the failings of the Health Service.

In the published report (1984) Griffiths proposed the introduction of general managers, who, in his view, would be able to lead services more cost-effectively. It was intended that key members of the disciplines they managed would professionally advise these managers. For the nursing profession this meant that line managers were no longer experienced nurses, which caused concern relating to professional issues and to the representation of community nursing views in policy making and community planning (Thornton 1995).

The introduction of general managers was followed in 1991 by internal market reforms. This step was intended to improve services by introducing competition and a purchaser–provider split. In theory, purchasers would 'shop around' for the best deal. General practice (GP) fund-holders were allocated an annual sum of money to buy a defined range of services for patients.

The mixed economy of health care was intended to restrain the bureaucracy of the 'nanny state' and increase input from voluntary and private organisations (Pierson 1998). The result was an increase in the amount of time and effort spent liaising with a great number of people, but it did also create opportunities for flexibility.

In May 1997 a large majority elected the Labour government to power under the leadership of Tony Blair – signalling the end of the long Conservative hold on government. Frank Dobson led a well-prepared team into the Department of Health. Policies began to be issued almost immediately (Hyde 2001). A key feature of the health policies of this Labour government was that they were 'joined up' with those of education and employment. In documents such as *Saving Lives: Our Healthier Nation* (DOH 1999), links between health and issues such as poverty, housing and employment

were acknowledged. Nurses, who daily witness the effects of these links, welcomed this approach.

The Labour government continued the work begun by the Conservative administration in shifting the balance of care delivery into the primary care sector, to create a primary care-led NHS. Within 9 months of Labour gaining office, *The New NHS: Modern, Dependable* (DOH 1997), a 10-year plan for health, had been published. This heralded the introduction of health improvement programmes (HIPs) and the development of primary care groups (PCGs) into primary care trusts (PCTs), which are, in effect, based around clusters of general practice surgeries. A major radical reform of the NHS was in prospect.

PCTs were fully established in England by April 2002. The equivalent bodies in Scotland are also called primary care trusts; in Wales they are known as local health boards; in Northern Ireland as local health and social care groups (Savage 2003). PCTs are responsible for assessing, planning and delivering health services, improving the health of the defined population, and working towards the proposed public health agenda (DOH 1999). They work collaboratively with local partners, such as Social Services, and the local community. Working alongside the PCTs, on a contractual basis, are the NHS trusts. The role of the health authorities has changed significantly: the recently formed strategic health authorities are larger organisations than the previous authorities, and provide overall management for both PCTs and NHS trusts. The equivalent organisations in other parts of the UK are: in Scotland, unified health boards; in Wales, health authorities; and, in Northern Ireland, health and social services boards (Savage 2003).

Alongside these structural changes, government policy focused on the needs of patients and their carers, and advocated patient participation in care (DOH 2001a). *A First Class Service: Quality in the New NHS* (DOH 1998) considered the quality of services offered, and launched clinical governance as a new framework for ensuring efficient and effective care within the NHS. Nurses were, on the whole, more receptive to the idea than their medical colleagues, who have traditionally monitored themselves. Many community nurses have taken the lead in issues of clinical governance. Quality is high on the agenda, and various structures are in place to ensure the optimum standards, including national service frameworks (NSFs), the National Institute for Clinical Excellence (NICE), and the Commission for Health Care Audit and Inspection (DOH 2000). In July 2000 the government published *The NHS Plan*, which sets the agenda for health care services centred on the patient and tailored to the patient's needs. The onus is on PCTs to implement national guidelines to meet the needs of their respective local communities.

The PCTs form the hub of the new NHS and are politically and financially powerful. Nurse representatives appointed to PCT boards need to be assertive, astute, have effective leadership skills and a clear vision of the future for community nursing.

CHALLENGES AND OPPORTUNITIES FOR COMMUNITY NURSING

The NHS Plan (DOH 2000) committed to the extension of nursing roles in all settings. The development of such initiatives as rapid response, intermediate care, early discharge and nurse-led clinics offer challenges and opportunities for community nurses. In 2001 the Department of Health published a report, *Shifting the Balance of Power*, which set out a programme of change designed to empower patients and the workforce to deliver this ambitious plan.

Politicians recognise the enormity of the task set before people and acknowledge that a huge cultural shift is necessary together with effective communication at all levels of the NHS organisation. Effective implementation of clinical governance is pivotal to the development of innovative community nursing practice and different ways of working. After more than 50 years of domination by the acute, specialist, hospital-based service, these changes are radical. *Liberating the Talents* (DOH 2002) calls for a transference of power to the front-line staff and – even more radically – to patients. There does seem to be a real attempt to change the status quo. So, it would appear that, after decades of being the Cinderella service, community health care has now gained a pivotal position in the NHS.

Community care and community nursing are by no means new phenomena. Looking back over time,

health care has been delivered in various ways and in a wide range of locations. The actual setting in which care occurs is directly influenced by the predominant form of health care at that time. This, in turn, develops as a result of the wider societal influences of the day (Tinson 1995).

Community nurses work in a great variety of settings – clinics, health centres, people's homes, schools, workplaces and private homes. Additionally, they work with different groups of people. For example, school nurses tend to focus upon children and adolescents and occupational health nurses care for a specified workforce. Some community nurses may care for all age groups, but spend much of their time with a particular subgroup. The majority of district nurse visits tend to be to older people (Audit Commission 1999). Community nurses work together with other team members. Collaboration and team working are essential for effective patient care. These issues are addressed in Chapter 6.

DEMOGRAPHIC ISSUES

The United Kingdom has been described as an ageing society, in which the number of people over the age of 80 years is set to increase by almost half as many again by 2025 and the number of people over 90 years of age is predicted to double (DOHb 2001). The needs of older people and their carers are often complex, and assessment of these requires a high level of knowledge and skill (Ryder 1997). Effective community care depends on the co-ordination and integration of health and social care.

To ensure that appropriate and effective health and social care is available for those older people who become frail or ill will become one of the community services' greatest challenges. It is equally important to acknowledge the great potential older people have to contribute towards communities and to encourage their participation in designing and developing services.

There are, of course, other groups of people who need to be considered carefully. It is important not to stereotype individuals, but planning to meet the needs of people with common characteristics can produce very effective initiatives. Good examples of these can be found in the government's 'Sure Start' strategy (DOE 1998).

A tool, which may be of great help in assessment of local needs, is a community profile. This can aid the identification of health needs and should involve the general public's viewpoint. Professional groups and less formal agencies may work together to produce a health needs assessment to assist in prioritising. These important issues are addressed in more detail in Chapters 3 and 10.

COMMUNITY SPECIALIST PRACTICE

Policy directives and patient choice, amongst other factors, have led to the development today of a primary care-focused NHS. According to Clarke (1999), community specialist practitioners work with individuals, families and communities towards the achievement of independence. Community nurses work within a network of complex processes in particular localities – not just in a different context from their colleagues in institutional or acute care settings. Community nursing involves much more than a change of location. From an exploration of the literature, it soon becomes apparent that the term 'community' itself is extremely difficult to define, as it can be interpreted in a variety of ways. Three commonly identified elements associated with 'community' are locality, solidarity and significance. In beginning to grasp the dynamic nature of a community, we must embrace all three elements and gain insight into the complex social relationships that exist between people, families and the community as they experience health and illness (Clarke 1999).

Community nursing is a fairly unique area of practice, embracing a philosophy of care that relates to primary, secondary and tertiary prevention, to a wide range of different interventions, and to health education (McMurray 1993). The 'client' can be an individual, family or community. Advanced clinical skills are required to fulfil the role of community specialist practitioner, including highly developed interpersonal skills, critical thinking, decision making, creative management and leadership, and a high degree of self-awareness (Clarke 1999). Each member of the community nursing team provides a valuable contribution to the delivery of high-quality effective care.

Nurses are now delivering care in a variety of different ways within the community, and new initiatives within primary care include walk-in centres and nurse-led personal medical services (PMS). Nurses are increasingly becoming the 'gatekeepers' of health services in the community. In general practice, the patient's first point of contact is often a nurse.

As their roles develop in response to the current NHS reforms, community nurses are required to expand their repertoire of skills and expertise. Earlier hospital discharges and more sophisticated treatment regimes mean that nurses are engaged in more technical and complex packages of care. 'Hospital at home' services, often co-ordinated by community specialist practitioners and their team, provide early hospital discharge for specific groups of patients – for example, those recovering from orthopaedic surgery. Many community hospitals provide respite care in nurse-led beds and 'rapid response' teams prevent hospital admissions, for example, for chest infections and stroke (Thomas 2000).

'Intermediate care' refers to 'that range of services designed to facilitate transition from hospital to home, and from medical dependence to functional independence, where the objectives of care are not primarily medical, the patient's discharge destination is anticipated and a clinical outcome of recovery (or restoration of health) is desired' (Steiner and Vaughan 1997).

Wade and Lees (2002) suggest that now is an ideal time for a review of current health care provision, with appropriate intermediate care services providing an opportunity for practice development which can incorporate interdisciplinary working and build bridges between the acute and community sectors. There is potential for a more needs-led and person-centred approach to care.

Intermediate care can be delivered in a variety of settings, including community hospitals, hospital at home schemes, community assessment and rehabilitation schemes, social rehabilitation schemes, and hospital hotels. An interdisciplinary approach is called for in which nurses, social services personnel, therapists and medical staff work together. Within the framework for nursing in primary care, nurses, midwives and health visitors have been given three core functions: first contact, continuing care and public health. Community nurses will have a key role in delivering this exciting agenda (DOH 2002). In conclusion, the following chapters further develop the issue raised in this Introduction.

REFERENCES

Audit Commission (1999) *First Assessment: A Review of District Nursing in England and Wales*. London: Audit Commission.

Clarke, J. (1999) Revisiting the concepts of community care and community health nursing. *Nursing Standard*, 14(10): 34–6.

Department of Education (1998) *Primary School League Tables*. London: The Stationery Office.

Department of Health (1997) *The New NHS: Modern, Dependable*. London: The Stationery Office.

Department of Health (1998) *A First Class Service: Quality in the New NHS*. London: The Stationery Office.

Department of Health (1999) *Saving Lives*. London: The Stationery Office.

Department of Health (2000) *The NHS Plan*. London: The Stationery Office.

Department of Health (2001a) *Shifting the Balance* DOH: London: The Stationery Office.

Department of Health (2001b) *National Service Framework for Older People*. London: The Stationery Office.

Department of Health (2001c) *The Expert Patient : A New Approach To Chronic Disease Management in the 21st Century*. London: The Stationery Office.

Department of Health (2002) *Liberating the Talents: Helping Primary Care Trusts and Nurses to Deliver the NHS Plan*. London: The Stationery Office.

Department of Health and Social Services (1977) *The Way Forward: Priorities in Health and Social Services*. London: HMSO.

Department of Health and Social Services (1983) *NHS Management Enquiry* (Chair: Sir Roy Griffiths). London: HMSO.

Hyde, V. (ed.) (2001) *Community Nursing and Health Care: Insights and Innovations*. London: Arnold.

Lawton, S., Cantrell, J. and Harris, J. (2000) *District Nursing: Providing Care in a Supportive Context*. London: Arnold.

McMurray, A. (1993) *Community Health Nursing: Primary Health Care in Practice*. London: Churchill Livingstone.

Pierson, C. (1998) *Beyond the Welfare State? The New Political Economy of Welfare* (2nd edn). Cambridge: Polity Press.

Ryder, E. (1997) Needs of older people. In S. Burley, E.E. Mitchell, K. Melling, M. Smith, S. Chilton and C. Crumplin, *Contemporary Community Nursing*. London: Arnold.

Savage, C. (2003) Where is the best place to nurse? *Nursing Times*, 99(10): 22–6.

Steiner A. and Vaughan, B. (1997) *Intermediate Care. A discussion paper arising from the King's Fund seminar held 30 October 1996*. London: King's Fund.

Thomas, S. (2000) The changing face of community nursing. *Primary Health Care*, 10(5): 21–4.

Thornton, C. (1995) The changing face of management. In P. Cain, V. Hyde and E. Howkins (eds), *Community Nursing: Dimensions and Dilemmas*. London: Arnold.

Tinson, S. (1995) Assessing health need: a community perspective. In P. Cain, V. Hyde and E. Howkins (eds), *Community Nursing: Dimensions and Dilemmas*. London: Arnold.

Wade, S. and Lees, L. (2002) The who, why, what of intermediate care. *Journal of Community Nursing* 16(10): 6–10.

2

New ways of working

Anne Smith

Learning outcomes

- Define the changing perception of service delivery in respect of the modernisation agenda.
- Examine the influence of the organisational culture on practice development.
- Identify new ways of working and delivering services in accordance with local targets.
- Analyse the need for skills development in leadership and management of change for practitioners at all levels.

Rapid changes have occurred within the NHS since the return of the Labour government to power in 1997. This commenced with *The New NHS: Modern, Dependable* (DOH 1997) and has been consolidated in *The NHS Plan* (DOH 2000a). Health and social policy have provided the driver for change and health care professionals have been required to respond. Clinical governance and quality issues (see DOH 1999d) have impacted on the organisation of the health service and the delivery of services. The aim of this chapter is to consider the effect of these changes. The focus of the discussion will be an analysis of how they have affected community care, and the new ways of working required to accommodate them.

delivery, and the focus is now on providing a patient-centred service based on local need (DOH 2000a), which is identified through exercises such as community profiling. There has been a conceptual shift away from illness orientation to health promotion (Naidoo and Wills 2000). There is a greater focus on the social aspects of people's lives that may affect their health. The individual, whilst being consulted over services, is also being expected to take some responsibility for his/her own health. However, it is recognised that health promotion strategies need to be targeted beyond the individual's behaviour, as the health of the general public is affected by many factors over which they have no personal control: for example, global warming and air pollution.

THE CHANGING PERCEPTION OF SERVICE DELIVERY

Previously the NHS has been service-led, with an authoritarian, 'top–down' approach. The medical model of health care has predominated (Burke 2001). In recent years there has been a paradigm shift in the underpinning philosophy of care

Exercise

Reflect on factors that affect your health over which you have no control. Consider your contribution to maintaining your local environment.

The government's commitment to supporting healthy living initiatives is demonstrated through the introduction of services such as smoking cessation clinics (DOH 1999b). This particular initiative has been placed within the remit of health visitors, district nurses and practice nurses. Their autonomy in this area has been further recognised by their being permitted to prescribe the relevant nicotine replacement therapy for the patients involved. Evidence suggests that this activity is one of the most influential health-promoting activities, and provides a measurable impact on health. The National Institute for Clinical Excellence has published guidelines to endorse this (2002). One example of a simple but effective innovation is described by Roberts (2002), who, in consultations, used three key questions to determine patients' readiness to give up smoking. The answers given by the patient indicate whether they are definitely resolved, or are considering 'quitting' but require more support to do so. This then enables the practitioner to arrange a suitable follow-up appointment to provide that support.

The new agenda is being directed by publications such as *The NHS Plan* (DOH 2000a) and *Shifting the Balance of Power* (DOH 2001a), which have evolved from *The NHS: Modern, Dependable* (1997). It will be influenced further by the forecasted demographic trends over the next 20 years – trends that have been substantiated in the 2001 census. This identified a greater proportion of the population being over the age of 60 than under 16 for the first time. The implications of this fact are enormous, together with the evidence that suggests that a quarter of the health care accessed during a person's life is accessed during the final years (Wanless 2001).

The infrastructure of the NHS has been radically altered. Primary care trusts (PCTs) have now emerged as the main provider of services. Revenue released from the Department of Health gives PCTs control of 75 per cent of the total health budget (DOH 2002b). Services are being delivered in innovative ways: for example, walk-in centres, NHS Direct. PCTs are now commissioning services at a local level, sensitive to the specific needs of their communities (DOH 2002b). Personal medical services (PMS) demonstrate this concept, and walk-in centres provide quick and effective access for clients, especially those who, because they are

working full-time, may have found surgery hours prohibitive.

> ## Exercise
>
> Consider what experience you or members of your family have as patients accessing these services.

These initiatives have also led to an expansion of nurse-led services, and the timely extension of nurse prescribing has enhanced nurses' contributions to this target. Other examples of innovations have been in operation over a longer period of time. 'Intermediate care' (DOH 2001b) is well established in many communities and offers a service that reduces pressure on acute beds, whilst meeting the needs of clients more effectively than previous arrangements, which were less flexible. This has provided the opportunity for targeting local problems with the appropriate services, building on previous initiatives evidenced by health action zones (HAZ) and health improvement programmes (HIPs) (DOH 1997). More recent publications (e.g. DOH 2002c) provide guidance on the priorities that local organisations are required to consider when planning future developments in community services. The main theme of this document echoes the underlying philosophy of service delivery in acknowledging the perspectives of all parties involved, including the patient. The public health agenda has also been emphasised, as each PCT is required to have a public health professional on the board. This emphasis is further demonstrated by the development of roles for health care professionals that are concerned with promoting public health. Within some community specialist nursing disciplines this has engendered a new conceptual base to the provision of services, particularly significant within the realms of school nursing and health visiting. Historically the school nursing service has been responsible for duties that have mimicked a medical model of care concerned with the completion of school medicals and health screening and surveillance. This image is swiftly changing, following the publication of *School Nursing: A National Framework for Practice* (CPHVA 2000), which identifies the school nurse as a dynamic member of the multi-disciplinary team, more involved than previously in issues of health promotion and education. A clear example of such innovation has been provided in *Liberating the Talents* (DOH 2002a), in which a school nurse describes her development of a profiling tool that identifies health and social issues within the school population so that these can be targeted to improve health.

It is increasingly obvious that the way that health care is delivered has been influenced by a shift in focus and this is common to all community disciplines. The practitioner's role is increasingly evolving as one with political and ethical dimensions. One clear example of the public's behaviour being affected by the media and their own interpretation of risk has been demonstrated through the MMR (measles, mumps and rubella) vaccination debate. Clinical staff were in a prime position to offer advice and influence behaviours. The health consequences resulting from the non-uptake of this vaccine were not clearly defined and therefore the public may not have been fully informed as to the implications of their decisions. The outcome has been that now there are unvaccinated infants susceptible to contracting these communicable diseases and the 'herd' immunity relied upon to control them is lost (Lewendon and Maconachie 2002). The public health issues underpinning this debate and the public health dimension that has become an expectation within every professional's remit will be explored further in Chapter 9.

Exercise

Reflect on how issues concerning a public health approach have influenced your own views of service delivery. Has it influenced the way that you work with your patients?

Currently practitioners are trying to understand and manage transition. New roles have been created, job descriptions reconfigured and employees are reorientating to their new responsibilities within the emerging structures. These events have taken place against a backdrop of quality enhancement and clinical governance (DOH 1999d). There is a focus on measuring and justifying the delivery of services whilst ensuring

that the patient's perspective is sought and documented (DOH 2002c). For those engaged in delivering services and providing continuity of care whilst all the reorganisation is occurring there is a sense of unease and instability. These behaviours can be clearly related to Tuckman's (1965) model of group life in which the group of individuals pass through several stages of 'forming' and 'storming' prior to settling into any type of team formation that is able to perform effectively.

However, it is an environment that can provide opportunities for those who feel enabled. Other practitioners may resist change by raising barriers to prevent any development being successful. These issues will be considered later, and coping strategies discussed.

Other major influences on the delivery of care are the monitoring procedures established to measure performance and the penalties incurred for failing to achieve targets. The National Institute for Clinical Excellence and the Commission for Health Improvement are both involved with ensuring quality in health care delivery underpinned by the implementation of research and evidence-based practice.

One key element of the new approach to the delivery of health care has been the emphasis on widening access. The changing perception therefore relates to both patients and staff as new initiatives are operationalised. The intention is that patients see a health service that is responding more appropriately to individual need and staff are increasingly aware that the provision of care is becoming more patient focused.

The new public health agenda has a strong emphasis on involving, inspiring and supporting local communities to undertake projects in which they, the public, propose and lead the changes (James and Barker 2001).

It may be useful to view this concept in relation to the principles of 'social marketing theory', first described by Kotler and Zaltman (1971, cited in Lefebvre 1992). Lefebvre's (1992) definition states that social marketing is 'a method of empowering people to be totally involved and responsible for their wellbeing: a problem-solving process that may suggest new and innovative ways to attack health and social problems. It is not social control.' The principles are adapted from a business base but have relevance to the introduction of health promoting behaviours from a micro and a macro perspective. (See Chapter 10 for further discussion of this concept.)

Exercise

What evidence are you aware of concerning patient participation in the decision making in your area? Identify examples of how these decisions have affected services.

THE ORGANISATIONAL CULTURE

Central to the notion of patient-centred care is the fact that a new approach is necessary. The structure of the whole organisation has been radically altered to facilitate this. Care cannot be delivered in a vacuum so the devolving of decision making and commissioning to localities should assist in the provision of services sensitive to local need (DOH 2002b).

However, these policy initiatives cannot be introduced without a consideration of the staff who will be implementing them. Many of the changes have already caused confusion as new roles have been established and new services developed. Sometimes this has been done without considering the services already in place. Poole (2002) advocates that real working in primary care necessitates an understanding of the complex issues involved. The nature of the work concerns investing in relationships and dealing with people who do not function in a predictable way like machines. Consequently staff must also adapt to the situations in which they find themselves and be aware of the loss of control that might be experienced. The authoritative or 'top–down' model of health care delivery has been succeeded by a more democratic, negotiated model. Poole offers some practical strategies for coping. She suggests that those delivering the services should invest time in developing relationships rather than focusing on roles and functions. Other essential considerations are flexibility in structuring working practice and, underpinning this, a sound communication system.

Community nurses are central to the delivery of the change process. The clinical governance agenda strongly influences working practice, with audit being an important component of practice. The nurses' contribution to the development of a 'new NHS' was documented in *Making a Difference* (DOH 1999a). This publication outlined the leadership qualities necessary to manage a swiftly changing service and initiated programmes such as the LEO (leading empowered organisations) programme to prepare nurses for their pivotal role (Garland, Smith and Faugier 2002).

A culture shift has also been experienced as budgets were amalgamated between health and social services. This was to promote the provision of a seamless service and to encourage integrated working, necessitating the removal of professional boundaries. One practical example of the Department of Health's commitment to such initiatives is the 'Single Assessment Process' outlined in *National Service Framework for the Older Person* (DOH 2001b). This has required professionals to co-operate in new ways to deliver appropriate care. Wild (2002) comments that a truly person-centred approach will only be achieved when professional boundaries have been dissolved.

Public service management styles require to be analysed in order to understand the philosophy underpinning the change of emphasis. The evolution of PCTs has ensured that the hierarchical and bureaucratic structures formally associated with health service management are becoming flatter and more democratic, with decisions being taken by those who are closer to the point of delivery and more aware of the outcomes.

The NHS bears little resemblance to the organisation it was even a decade ago. Confusion persists over the new structural components and role definitions. Job titles appear creative and expansive as boundaries and expectations have not been clearly identified. 'Skill mix' has become a term encompassing innovative strategies to develop members of the workforce to enable them to offer support in a variety of ways; for example receptionists who are also trained as phlebotomists and ECG (electrocardiogram) technicians.

Localities operate in very different ways, and moving from one area to another can provide a culture shock in itself. The sense of change in the organisational culture is devolved to a very personal level. However, the reorganisation of community care is a constant feature throughout. The drivers for change are also similar, but the interpretation of how the agenda will be met may vary enormously according to the location in which the care is delivered.

> ## Exercise
>
> Consider which government initiatives have been implemented in your locality.

NEW WAYS OF WORKING

The NHS Plan (DOH 2000a) has outlined a 10-year plan of investment and reform in order to modernise the NHS. The workforce is central to that plan. As previously noted, the NHS must acknowledge that a culture shift is required. Bureaucratic management concentrating on service provision dictated by resource allocation is no longer acceptable. A dynamic and flexible approach is advocated, which places the emphasis on patient participation in decision making. This approach must be transparent, and a variety of options have been developed to facilitate this.

The introduction of local patient forums and the formation of patient advisory liaison services (PALS) indicate that the public are being consulted (Chapman 2002). Collaborative working must be embraced in its widest sense – to include the recipient of care. Further evidence of the government's commitment is clearly demonstrated by the introduction of the white paper *The Expert Patient* (DOH 2001c). Whilst acknowledging that many patients with chronic diseases have a more in-depth knowledge of the personal management of their particular condition than the professional, it also conveys the message that patients are able to be more independent if encouraged to take control of the management. This relates to the theory described by Rotter (1954) concerning 'locus of control'. It is also aligned to the concept prevalent in the government documents that the patient should remain in control of the decisions about their health and treatment.

Health promotion strategies to prevent the onset of chronic diseases such as coronary heart disease and diabetes are also advocated. Again the government's commitment to this has been demonstrated by the publication of national service frameworks, for example DOH 2000c and 2001b, which prescribe standards, respectively, for the care of individuals suffering from coronary heart disease, and for the care of older patients, in order to provide equity of care throughout the country. Integral to these frameworks are initiatives concerned with providing both primary and secondary prevention. An example of responding with a team approach is quoted by Fairhead (2003), who describes how a community mental health nurse worked alongside a practice nurse to develop her expertise in managing patients with depression. The general practitioners and patients gave a very positive response, when surveyed, to the resulting improvement in services.

New ways of working are emerging in response to the demographic influences within the workforce. The shortage of nurses is already apparent, and is set to get worse, particularly as the profile of community nurses indicates an ageing population. The problem was identified in 1999 (DOH 1999a) and a response by the government was to provide more training places. However this was not sufficient to resolve the problem. Other solutions have been considered, various of them initiated by the document *A Health Service for All Talents* (DOH 2000b). Cadet schemes have been reinstated. Further incentives have been provided for those workers (health care assistants) with NVQ qualifications to undertake more in-depth training. These schemes are supported by their employers and delivered in the workplace environment whilst they continue with their employment. This has several advantages in that the workforce is not depleted whilst the care assistants are training and they continue to receive a salary whilst extending their knowledge and skills. Once trained, their employment status will be enhanced to that of 'assistant practitioners'. They will also qualify academically with a foundation degree (Greater Manchester Workforce Development Confederation 2002). The intention is to initiate a 'skills escalator', which practitioners will be able to 'step on' and 'step off', to provide flexible learning and training, accessible to all individuals at all grades (DOH 2003).

The government has pledged its commitment to initiatives to educate the workforce and support life-long learning for all sectors of the workforce, and such initiatives as this demonstrate the commitment.

Exercise

Consider the skill mix of the team in which you work. What sort of roles do the members of the team adopt? Are people adopting different roles? Is the team delivering services in a different way? Are the patients seeking the service for different reasons than they were two years ago?

Flexible working is further enhanced by 'family-friendly policies' advocated in such documents as *Improving Working Lives* (DOH 2002d) The emphasis is on recruiting and retaining staff by offering working hours that complement domestic responsibilities.

As previously discussed, the different community disciplines are challenged by a variety of demands according to their roles, although some issues are common to all. This is considered within specialist practitioner degree courses. All community nursing professionals are educated within a core course which includes a specialist element to reflect their specific discipline. This demonstrates the value placed on all these professionals' contributions to the primary health care team in fulfilling the health improvement agenda.

The NHS Plan (DOH 2000a) placed great emphasis on the development of integrated teams and this was to include practice nurses, who historically have been set apart from their community nursing colleagues due to their employment contracts with GPs. In many instances these arrangements are changing following the formation of PCTs.

New ways of working and managing care are continually being influenced by advances in technology and the health service's attempt to embrace them. Examples of such influences are the increasing use of telemedicine and the computerisation of patient records. The improvement in communication provided by these systems with their ability to transfer information, particularly between hospitals, laboratories and surgeries has an impact on patient care.

KEY SKILLS FOR LEADERSHIP AND MANAGEMENT OF CHANGE

The community environment is changing beyond recognition and there is a requirement for practitioners to change their ways of working to manage it. Practice development can be achieved in many different ways and the success of it depends on the management of change. As previously stated, examples of innovative schemes have been published in the document *Liberating the Talents* (DOH 2002a). This publication describes creative ways in which health care can be delivered, acknowledging the fact that 90 per cent of patient journeys involve a contact in primary care (O'Dowd 2002).

Unsworth (2001) contends that within the NHS professionals are expected to plan and implement change in practice, often with very little support. Business organisations meanwhile will import experts to manage the change process. These approaches to managing change refer to 'external' or 'internal' change agents (Broome 1998).

However, change management is a complex process for which practitioners need adequate preparation. The requirement for preparation was clearly identified in *Making a Difference* (DOH 1999a) and reinforced in the recommendations of *The NHS Plan* (DOH 2000a), in which nurses were proposed as the main implementers of the new agenda in practice. A national nursing leadership project, initiated by the Department of Health, is providing training for those considered best placed to move practice forward, advocating an empowering approach. Well established in this area is the LEO (Leading an Empowered Organisation) programme (Garland, Smith and Faugier 2002).

The Department of Health has invested in a variety of measures to ensure that leadership training is devolved to all levels of staff, since leadership qualities do not necessarily only exist within those staff in positions of seniority. Clinical 'change agents' do not need to be team leaders but any practitioner who is supported to change practice.

Exercise

Visit the nursing leadership website and explore the educational opportunities that it offers at www.nursingleadership.co.uk.

Certain approaches need to be considered if change is going to be effective and smoothly implemented. A primary consideration is that of planning the change and providing a sound rationale for the need to change. If this is clearly articulated and agreed by the team members the chances of success are more likely.

The nature of current change is that it is government-led and -driven, which means that it is difficult for the practitioner to see the need for change or take responsibility for it. This often leads to resistance and hostility. It is vital to consider the perceived benefits of change. SWOT analysis is a useful exercise that will help practitioners do this (Adams 2000). It involves compiling a list of statements that identify the effects of the change under four headings: strengths, weaknesses, opportunities and threats. It must be remembered that the type of change mainly associated with the new arrangements is 'imposed change', often unplanned and swiftly introduced, and with those people who will be most affected are not being consulted over the best means of implementation. Unless SWOT analysis shows obvious benefits to all concerned, practitioners will continue to lack enthusiasm and motivation.

It is clear that change cannot be effectively managed unless certain procedures are followed to identify the need for it: for example, audit, research, reflection, SWOT analysis (Adams 2000). These provide the evidence for change, after which planning the change process must be undertaken. If the ideas of those who will be involved are incorporated, or their comments sought, they are more likely to support rather than resist the change. 'Planned change' is generally better received and more likely to succeed than 'unplanned change' (Broome 1998).

It is worthwhile pausing here to consider the components of change management theory discussed by Lewin (1951), as these underpin any strategy that may be devised to manage change in the working environment. Lewin describes a three-stage approach: unfreezing, moving (or changing) and refreezing. The unfreezing stage concerns recognising that a change is necessary. This need may be identified through reflective practice or examining research that promotes different ways of working. The change requires planning in order to achieve the proposed outcomes. Finally, once the change has been implemented refreezing occurs as the new practice is adopted. As with any new initiatives there will be those who are motivated to change and those who are cynical and less keen; enthusiasts ready to accept and implement change; but equally 'laggards', who are difficult to convince. Managing these 'laggards' is the real challenge, and the leadership style of the person who is facilitating the change is relevant to success. Styles of leadership vary according to the character of the individual and their position in the organisation.

The above is an extremely simplified explanation of the change management process. In reality, the successful implementation of a change in practice is a complex task.

Mulhall's text (1999) examines various theoretical perspectives. Ultimately however, the culture of the practice environment has a strong determining influence on whether the change is effectively introduced and adopted. Therefore practice development is the remit of all staff, and to achieve success in this area requires an inclusive approach, in which everyone feels they can contribute.

CONCLUSION

It is necessary and indeed the responsibility of all NHS employees, in order to meet the demands placed upon them, to become involved in providing a service that sets the patient at the centre. It is also important that health professionals are responsive to the feedback offered by the patient (Hollins 2002). If the targets of the NSFs are to be met, practice innovation and new ways of working are required in which individuals are empowered to be self-supporting in taking responsibility for their personal health and wellbeing and that of their community. Models of community health practice (Chalmers and Kristajanson 1989) and practice development (Page 2002) can provide a framework for this activity.

The community nurse's role is multi-faceted and the approach must be adaptable in order to respond to the variety of caring, supportive, or pro-active roles that she may be required to adopt in this diverse area.

The Chief Nursing Officer summed up the diverse roles of primary health care practitioners when briefing PCT lead nurses:

> It isn't just what you do that matters, it is also how you work that is important – putting the patient and community first, empowering front line staff and working in partnership across health and social care.

(Mullally 2002)

FURTHER READING

Iles, V. and Sutherland, K. (2001) *Managing Change in the NHS. Organisational Change: A Review for Health Care Managers, Professionals and Researchers.* London: National Co-ordinating Centre for NHS Delivery and Organisation R and D.

Mulhall, A. (1999) *Changing Practice: The Theory. Nursing Times Clinical Monograph No 2.* London: Nursing Times Books.

Rink, E. (2000) *Integrated Nursing Teams in Primary Care. Nursing Times Clinical Monograph No 49.* London: Nursing Times Books.

REFERENCES

Adams, C. (2000) *Clinical Effectiveness: A Practical Guide for Nurses.* London: Community Practitioners and Health Visitors Association.

Broome, A. (1998) *Managing Change.* London: Macmillan.

Burke, W. (2001) Can you feel the force? The importance of power in practice development. In S. Spencer, J. Unsworth and W. Burke (eds), *Developing Community Nursing Practice.* Buckingham: Open University.

Chalmers, K. and Kristajanson, L. (1989) The theoretical basis for nursing at the community level: a comparison of three models. *Journal of Advanced Nursing*, 14: 569–74.

Chapman, L. (2002) Involving patients in the new NHS. *Primary Health Care*, 12(21): 10–12.

Community Practitioners and Health Visitors Association (2000) *School Nursing: A National Framework for Practice.* London: CPHVA.

Department of Health (1997) *The New NHS: Modern, Dependable.* London: The Stationery Office.

Department of Health (1998) *A First Class Service: Quality in the New NHS.* London: The Stationery Office.

Department of Health (1999a) *Making a Difference: Strengthening the Nursing, Midwifery and Health Visiting Contribution to Health and Health Care.* London: The Stationery Office.

Department of Health (1999b) *Smoking Kills.* London: The Stationery Office.

Department of Health (1999c) *Sure Start.* London: The Stationery Office.

Department of Health (1999d) *Clinical Governance: Quality in the New NHS.* London: The Stationery Office.

Department of Health (2000a) *The NHS Plan: A Plan for Investment, A Plan for Reform.* London: The Stationery Office.

Department of Health (2000b) *A Health Service for All Talents: Developing the Workforce.* London: The Stationery Office.

Department of Health (2000c) *National Service Framework for Coronary Heart Disease.* London: The Stationery Office.

Department of Health (2001a) *Shifting the Balance of Power: The Next Steps.* London: The Stationery Office.

Department of Health (2001b) *National Service Framework for Older People.* London: The Stationery Office.

Department of Health (2001c) *The Expert Patient: A New Approach to Chronic Disease Management in the 21st Century.* London: The Stationery Office.

Department of Health (2002a) *Liberating the Talents.* London: The Stationery Office.

Department of Health (2002b) *Delivering the NHS Plan.* London: The Stationery Office. And see: www.doh.gov.uk/deliveringthenhsplan/index/htm

Department of Health (2002c) *Improvement, Expansion and Reform: The Next Three Years.* London: The Stationery Office. And see: http://www.doh.gov.uk/planning2003-2006/improvementexpansionreform.pdf

Department of Health (2002d) *Improving Working Lives for the Allied Health Professions and Health Care Scientists.* London: The Stationery Office.

Department of Health (2003*) Human Resources Skills Escalator. London:* The Stationery Office. And see: www.doh.gov.ukhrinthenhs/section4b/skillsescalatorhomepage.htm

Fairhead, C. (2003) A new role in managing depression. *Primary Health Care*, 13(21): 18–20.

Garland, G., Smith, S. and Fuagier, J. (2002) Supporting clinical leaders in achieving organisational change. *Professional Nurse*,17(8): 490–2.

Greater Manchester Workforce Development Confederation (2002) *Developing the Modern Workforce: Annual Report 2001/2002.* See: www.gmconfed.org.uk

Hollins, M. (2002) The opportunity for nurses to manage themselves. *Primary Health Care,* 12(4): 10–12.

Hyde, V. and Cotter, C. (2001) The development of community nursing in the light of the NHS Plan. In V. Hyde (ed.), *Community Nursing and Health Care: Insights and Innovations.* London: Arnold.

Iles, V. and Sutherland, K. (2001) *Managing Change in the NHS. Organisational Change: A Review for Health Care Managers, Professionals and Researchers.* London: National Co-ordinating Centre for NHS Delivery and Organisation R and D.

James, T. and Barker, E. (2001) Community development. In D. Sines, F. Appleby and E. Raymond (eds), *Community Health Care Nursing* (2nd edn). Oxford: Blackwell Science.

Lefebvre, C. (1992) Social marketing and health promotion. In R. Bunton and G. Macdonald (eds), *Health Promotion. Disciplines and Diversity.* London: Routledge.

Lewendon, G. and Maconachie, M. (2002) Why are children not being immunised? Barriers and risks to immunisation uptake in South Devon. *Health Education Journal,* 61(3): 212–20.

Lewin, K. (1951) *Field Theory in Social Science.* New York: Harper & Row.

Mulhall, A. (1999) *Changing Practice: The Theory. Nursing Times Clinical Monographs No 2.* London: Nursing Times Books.

Mullally S. (2002) *Special Edition: Chief Nursing Officer Bulletin July 2002.* And see: www.doh.gov.uk/cno/pctbulletinspecialjuly02.htm

Naidoo, J. and Wills, J. (2000) *Health Promotion: Foundations for Practice* (2nd edn). Edinburgh: Baillière Tindall in association with the Royal College of Nursing.

National Health Service Centre for Research and Dissemination (1999) *Effective Health Care Bulletin,* 5(1): 9–14. And see: www.york.ac.uk/inst/crd

National Institute for Clinical Excellence (2002) *Guidance on the Use of Nicotine Replacement Therapy (NRT) and Bupropion for Smoking Cessation.* Technology Appraisal Guidance No 39.

O'Dowd, A. (2002) The primary care revolution. *Nursing Times,* 98(47): 1–11.

Page, S. (2002) The role of practice development in modernising the NHS. *Nursing Times,* 98(11): 34–6.

Poole, J. (2002) Complexity in primary care. *Primary Health Care,* 12(1): 16–17.

Roberts, J. (2002) Kicking the habit. *Primary Health Care,* 12(9): 27–32.

Rotter, J. (1954) Generalised expectations for internal v. external control and reinforcement. *Psychological Monographs,* 80.

Tuckman B. (1965) Developmental sequences in small groups. *Psychological Bulletin,* 63: 384–99.

Unsworth, J. (2001) Managing the development of practice. In S. Spencer, J. Unsworth and W. Burke (eds), *Developing Community Nursing Practice.* Buckingham: Open University.

Wanless, D. (2001) *Securing our Future Health : Taking a Long-term View.* London: HM Treasury.

Wild, D. (2002) The single assessment process. *Primary Health Care,* 12(1): 20–1.

Woodward, V. (2001) Evidence-based practice, clinical governance and community nurses. In V. Hyde (ed.), *Community Nursing and Health Care: Insights and Innovations.* London: Arnold.

3

Nursing in a community environment

Sue Chilton

Learning outcomes

- Discuss environmental, social, economic and political factors influencing the delivery of community health care services.
- Differentiate between a demand-driven and a needs-led approach to community health care service provision.
- Explain ways in which local services aim to be responsive to the specific needs of their population.
- Describe the role and key responsibilities of the eight community specialist practitioner nursing disciplines.
- Identify those mechanisms which need to be in place to ensure services are effective and efficient.

This chapter considers the context in which community nurses practise, and addresses the wide range of factors that impact upon the services they provide for patients. Demand-driven and needs-led services are compared, and ways of tailoring provision of care to fit local need are discussed. The roles and responsibilities of the eight community specialist practice disciplines are outlined and the key strategies for ensuring high-quality care are identified.

FACTORS INFLUENCING THE DELIVERY OF COMMUNITY HEALTH CARE SERVICES

Community nurses face many challenges within their evolving roles. The transition from working in an institutional setting to working in the community can be quite demanding at first. As a student on community placement or a newly employed staff nurse, it soon becomes apparent that there is a wide range of factors influencing the planning and delivery of community health care services. Within the home/community context, the issues that impact upon an individual's health are more apparent. People are encountered in their natural habitats rather than being isolated within the hospital setting. Assessment is so much more complex in the community as the nurse must consider the interconnections between the various elements of a person's lifestyle.

Exercise

Make a list of all those factors that might have an impact upon a person's health. It might be helpful to think about it on different levels: individual/family factors, community factors and societal/governmental factors.

Defining health is complex as it involves multiple factors. According to Blaxter (1990), health can be defined from four different perspectives: an absence of disease, fitness, ability to function and general wellbeing. The concept of health has many dimensions: physical, mental, emotional, social, spiritual and societal. All aspects of health are interdependent in an holistic approach. It is prudent to view an individual within the context of their wider socio-economic situation when considering issues relating to their health. There are acknowledged inequalities in health status between different people within society and major determinants include social class, culture, occupation, income, gender and geographical location. The Acheson report (1998), which informs the present national public health agenda, provides a fairly comprehensive review of the literature/research available on inequalities in health.

DOH (1998a) summarises some of the factors influencing health as follows:

- Fixed: genes, sex.
- Social and economic: poverty, employment and social exclusion.
- Environmental: air quality, housing, water quality, social environment.
- Lifestyle: diet, physical activity, smoking, alcohol, sexual behaviour and drugs.
- Access to services: education, NHS, Social Services, transport and leisure.

These different categories of influences upon health can be particularly useful in providing prompts when considering the health status of a local population of people.

Dahlgren and Whitehead (1991) present a comprehensive model consisting of four levels:

- Level 1: General socio-economic, cultural and environmental conditions.
- Level 2: Living and working conditions – housing, health care services, water and sanitation, unemployment, work environment, education, agriculture and food production.
- Level 3: Social and community networks.
- Level 4: Individual lifestyle factors.

The authors state that all four levels impact upon the health status of the individual, for whom age, sex and hereditary factors are also significant.

The increased emphasis lately on the development of a primary care-led NHS has come about in response to demographic, technological, political and financial influences amongst others. An increasing population of older people, shorter hospital stays, improvements in technology and patient preference have all contributed to the movement of resources from the acute to the primary care sector. The development of new competencies to provide services away from hospital settings (Thomas 2000) means that an increasing number of people with both acute and chronic conditions will eventually receive care at home or in a range of other locations within the community. It is envisaged that hospitals will mainly provide diagnostic and specialist services in the future.

HEALTH NEEDS ASSESSMENT

A quote from *Community-oriented Primary Care* summarises the principles underpinning a needs-led, as opposed to a demand-led, service:

Needs assessment requires more than epidemiological data on geographically defined populations. To be responsive to users, it requires the involvement of front-line service providers, particularly those based in the community. These information sources are complementary, and both need to be integrated to plan and deliver appropriate health services. Linking rigorous needs assessment to service definition and the iterative cycle of service assessment and revision requires close collaboration between commissioners and providers. Primary care professionals are closer to service users than most other providers, and have a key role in identifying health care needs.

Primary health care teams (PHCTs) are being required to assess their practice populations' needs to guide practice and to achieve targets in areas such as health promotion. Systematic approaches to these tasks are required.

Primary care organisations of the future will have to retain their capacity to provide quality personal care and develop a population orientation if they are to move from a demand-led service – however responsive – to needs-led practice, and a better integration of primary health care, secondary care, social services and the voluntary sector.

(King's Fund 1994: p.1)

This approach to primary health care is just as relevant today, particularly as we are now providing services to defined populations within primary care trust (PCT) boundaries. It is clearly important that we consider the actual/potential needs of our given population – regardless of our discipline – if we are to provide services that are relevant and efficient.

Example

An occupational health nurse working in a factory that produces chemicals may engage in health checks for new employees and respond to staff health problems on a daily basis. In addition, however, he/she might take part in screening activities with employees in order to identify potential physical/psychological health problems related to the nature of the work in question.

Bradshaw's taxonomy of need (1972), which describes four types of need, provides a useful starting point when addressing this subject: (1) 'normative' need is need as defined by professionals; (2) 'felt' need is a want as perceived by the population; (3) an 'expressed' need is a demand for a felt need to be met; and (4) a comparative need is defined by comparing services provided to individuals/populations with similar characteristics. In order for services to target needs appropriately, they need to respond to felt and expressed needs rather than normative need. Providing 'needs-led' services can be somewhat challenging for community nurses as it may well involve a greater empowerment of the client and a willingness on the part of the community nurse to re-examine their own motives/reasons for providing the current service in the way they do. This may lead to a fairly major change in the organisation of the service for the future, which will require regular evaluations.

In a review of the district nursing services across England and Wales, the Audit Commission (1999) recognised that at least one in ten referrals to district nurses (DNs) are inappropriate. It is recommended that DNs define more clearly the service they provide. One of the major reasons for inappropriate referrals appears to be a misunderstanding on the part of colleagues within the primary health care team regarding the role and the responsibilities of DNs. In response, DNs could address this issue in a number of ways.

Example

A district nursing team working within a particular locality of a PCT might decide to actively market their service. They may produce guidelines for referral (for GPs, hospital staff, other professional colleagues and patients/families). Service aims/objectives would reflect the needs of their specific client group (felt/expressed need) and not be based solely on normative need. Comparisons with other DN service guidelines might be carried out (comparative need) but variations in the characteristics of the different populations would need to be taken into account.

Community nurses can identify the needs of their given population by conducting a health needs assessment, which is a process of gathering information from a variety of sources in order to assist the planning and development of services. As society is constantly changing, health needs assessment is not a static exercise. According to the extract from *Community-oriented Primary Care* (King's Fund 1994) quoted above, data is required regarding disease patterns (epidemiology) and public health in a particular area (PCT or locality within PCT), as well as information regarding local environmental factors/resources (knowledge base/experience of community service providers). In other words, a combination of 'hard' (statistical/research-based/quantitative) data and 'soft' (experiential/anecdotal/qualitative) data.

Example

Consider the area/team in which you are working at present. What sources of information would help to inform you regarding the specific needs of your client group/population. Make a list and try to divide the information into either 'hard' or 'soft' data.

In capturing the 'essence' of a locality, the term 'community profile' is frequently used to describe an area in relation to its amenities, demography (characteristics of the population), public services, employment, transport and environment. Traditionally, health visitors, in particular, have been required to produce community profiles as a form of assessment during their training.

Any attempt to analyse the series of complex processes that make up a living community without the participation of local residents/consumers is a fairly fruitless exercise. In gathering information from a large community population, a variety of methods may prove useful. An approach known as participatory rapid appraisal has been described elsewhere (Chilton and Barnes 1997) and involves community members in the collection of information and in decision making related to this information. Originally used in developing countries to assess need within poor rural populations, it has been employed in deprived urban areas (Cresswell 1992). A wide variety of data collection methods are used and participatory rapid appraisal involves local agencies and organisations working together. By working in partnership with local residents, action is taken by community members who have identified issues of local concern/interest and discussed potential solutions. Clearly, participatory rapid appraisal could be used to help tackle specific issues as well as large-scale assessments.

Example

In a PCT, the local health improvement programme (HIP) target is to reduce teenage pregnancies. A participatory rapid appraisal approach to the issue might involve pregnant teenagers, health visitors, school nurses, school teachers, practice nurses, midwives, family planning clinic personnel, local hospital maternity services etc. Following government guidelines in the form of the Social Exclusion Unit's report (1999) on teenage pregnancies, data collection methods could include semi-structured interviews with key individuals, focus group interviews, written reports and hard data. By working together with teenagers who are pregnant in an appraisal of their needs, professionals may develop greater understanding of the key issues. A more co-ordinated approach to the challenge of reducing teenage pregnancies may be developed, which might necessitate changes to the responsibilities of the different disciplines involved. In promoting a collaborative initiative such as this, there is a greater awareness of the roles of other colleagues and duplication can be avoided.

MEETING THE NEEDS OF THE LOCAL POPULATION

Current government policy (DOH 1997, 2000a, 2001) stresses the importance of a localised approach to community health care service provision. Each PCT is different in terms of its characteristics, which might include its demography, geographical location, environment, amenities, transport systems, unemployment levels, deprivation scores, work opportunities and access to services, for example. As a result of these potential variations, it is important to interpret national guidelines according to local needs. Each PCT has its own individualised local targets for public health identified within a HIP and tailored to the specific requirements of the local population. Such targets are usually chosen following an examination of local information sources, such as epidemiological data collected by the public health department within the health authority, general practice (GP) profiles and caseload analysis data obtained from local health care practitioners.

By systematically reviewing local information sources and working within government/professional guidelines, community specialist practitioners have an opportunity to develop practice and more collaborative ways of working.

Example

From GP profile information, one locality within a PCT identified a significantly high percentage of the older population with dementia. As a result, the community psychiatric nurse team working with older people in the locality liaised with the practice nurses across the identified GP practices with a view to discussing the provision of support for the carers involved.

DOH (2001) highlights the importance of front-line staff taking responsibility for implementing many of the recent changes in the NHS. This will involve community nurses becoming more actively involved in health needs assessment. It has been recognised that there are populations whose health care needs are unmet (Latimer and Ashburner 1997), which presents community nurses with the challenge of redefining their services to more accurately respond to the needs of their particular patient group. Traditionally, many community nurses have responded to referrals, which are frequently inappropriate and often do not represent the most urgent needs of the population in terms of priority.

Responding more appropriately is not any easy task, as many of these unmet needs often require seeking out and might exist within the more disadvantaged sectors of society. It is not unreasonable to assume that many community nurses will require a greater understanding of different cultural issues and social value systems before they are able to identify specific unmet needs. The inverse care law means that, ironically, the more advantaged people in society tend to receive better health care services (Acheson report, 1998). Current NHS policy is attempting to rectify this anomaly and end the so-called 'postcode lottery', which suggests that health status can be determined on the basis of where a person lives.

Although national service frameworks (NSFs) are national guidelines produced to encourage the dissemination of best practice in relation to particular conditions or client groups, it is the responsibility of front-line staff to implement them locally and interpret them according to local conditions.

Exercise

In relation to the locality in which you are based in the community, find out about ways in which the NSFs are being implemented at a local level. Gather information regarding local initiatives and examples of any community nurses working in collaboration with other individuals/organisations/agencies in addressing the NSF guidelines.

Ensuring that local NHS organisations work together with local authorities, especially with regard to social care, is fundamental to the new ways of working, and PCTs are in an ideal position to facilitate this collaborative approach.

Clearly, there are differences between PCTs in terms of the locations in which community health care services are offered to patients. Provision will vary considerably between a rural and an urban PCT. For example, in a rural location, there might tend to be more community hospitals, providing accessible local services

that are not of a specialist nature, whereas walk-in centres, for example, tend to be located in more densely populated locations, such as city centres and airports.

In order to provide high-quality care to patients, community nurses need the necessary skills, knowledge and expertise and it is the responsibility of individual practitioners and their employing authority to ensure that the appropriate training is organised. Working alongside their local workforce confederation, PCTs or other employing authorities plan for the future recruitment and training of new staff and the continuing professional development of existing staff. PCTs will also develop and update policies and procedures in relation to the clinical responsibilities of community nurses and these should relate to the latest benchmarking criteria and government/professional guidelines.

Under the present government, it is suggested that patients should have an influence on the provision of health care services. Patients' views should therefore be considered by board members of the PCT, who are charged with the responsibility of ensuring patient participation.

COMMUNITY HEALTH CARE NURSING DISCIPLINES

A new understanding of community care as 'process' rather than 'context' is proposed by Clarke (1999) to enable us to value community nursing as advanced specialist practice in its own right, rather than as institutional or acute care nursing in another setting. Eng et al. (1992) encourage an 'understanding that a community is a 'living' organism with interactive webs of ties among organisations, neighbourhoods, families and friends'.

Community nursing takes place in a wide variety of settings.

Exercise

List as many different locations as you can where community nurses provide care. This might help you to identify particular client groups and go on to name some of the eight community specialist practice disciplines identified by the UK Central Council (UKCC) in 1994.

Recent government reforms in terms of the structures and systems that form the NHS (e.g. DOH 1997, 2000a, 2001) have led to an acknowledgement by community specialist practitioners that their roles and responsibilities need to be examined and redefined in preparation for the new challenges ahead. Leadership, practice development and partnership working are key elements within the roles of all community specialist practitioners (DOH 2001). The Nursing and Midwifery Council (NMC) are currently attempting to redefine the role of the specialist practitioner. In the early 1990s, the UKCC conducted the PREP (post-registration education and practice) project to clarify the future training requirements for post-registration nurses. At the time, eight community specialist practice disciplines were identified: occupational health nursing, community paediatric nursing, community learning disability nursing, community mental health nursing, general practice nursing, school nursing, health visiting and district nursing.

The UKCC (1994) proposed a common core-centred course for all specialities, which was to be at first degree level at least, and one year in length. According to the UKCC, the remit of community specialist practice embraces 'clinical nursing care, risk identification, disease prevention, health promotion, needs assessment and a contribution to the development of public health services and policy'. It is perhaps particularly pertinent in the current context of partnership working that we embrace those common aspects of our practice as community specialist practitioners. In espousing the uniqueness of the individual disciplines, there is an acknowledged danger that nurses will miss out on opportunities to influence a primary care-led NHS (Quinney and Pearson 1996)

Occupational health nursing (OHN)

OHN is a relatively new nursing discipline that has developed from its origins in 'industrial nursing' in the mid-19th century, when the role was mainly curative rather than preventative (Chorley 2001).

Occupational health nurses work within the wider occupational health services and play a preventive role in advising employers, employees and their representatives on health and safety issues in the working environment, and the adaptation of the working environment to the capabilities of the employees (RCN 1991).

The role of the OHN is concerned with preventing ill health which affects the ability to work, and ill health caused by employment, and also with promoting good health and developing health promotion strategies in the workplace. OHNs' responsibilities are as varied as the industries/businesses in which they are employed.

Chorley (2001) identifies five elements of the OHN role as being professional, managerial, business, environmental and educational responsibilities.

Many factors influence the future role of the OHN, including political, economic and public health care strategies. However, Chorley (2001) argues that OHNs can professionally influence key areas of their practice by assessing future health care trends through analysing research, reviewing epidemiological data and conducting needs assessment.

Community children's nursing (CCN)

According to the Royal College of Nursing (RCN 2002b), the past few decades have seen considerable growth and innovation for CCN services. In 1987, there was a total of 25 services in the UK; currently, there is a total of 150 CCN teams in England alone. There are very few areas (mainly rural) without a service.

The development of the CCN services has been supported by a number of pertinent reports (DOH 1991; DOH/NHSE 1996, Audit Commission 1993). The Department of Health and the NHS Executive (1996) agree that 'CCN services should be led, and predominantly staffed, by nurses who possess both registrations as a children's nurse and experience of community nursing'.

There are three key elements within the delivery of CCN services: (1) first contact/acute assessment, diagnoses, treatment and referral of children; (2) continuing care, chronic disease management and meeting the imperatives of the Children's NSF; and (3) public health/health protection and promotion programmes – working with children and families to improve health and reduce the impact of illness and disability (DOH 2002).

Community learning disability nursing (CLDN)

According to Barr (2001), there was a recognition of the need for more community-based services to be provided for people with learning disabilities living at home and their families in the mid-1970s. Around this time, different models of service were developing around the notion of 'normalisation', which is the underlying philosophy of many of the services provided for people with learning disabilities. Normalisation may be defined as 'a complex system which sets out to value positively devalued individuals and groups' (Race 1999).

Service principles for learning disability services should be based on an individual's assessed needs; flexible and sensitive in service provision; equitable and integrated with an accessible range of services that offer priority to those in the greatest need; prompt, effective and comprehensive and evaluated by the degree to which they provide privacy, dignity, independence, rights and fulfilment for people with learning disabilities (DHSS 1995).

CLDNs often work closely with other members of the multidisciplinary team. Bollard and Jukes (1999) stress the importance of CLDNs clarifying their working relationships with other community specialist practitioners and members of the primary health care team in order that people with learning disabilities do not fall between services or receive conflicting advice.

Community mental health nursing (CMHN)

The CMHN service has been well documented since its inception in the mid-1950s. The expertise of the CMHN lies in assessing the mental health of an individual within a family and social context. CMHNs may be located in health centres, GP practices, voluntary organisations and accident and emergency departments. They represent people with mental health needs and provide high quality therapeutic care (Long 2001). Four elements underpin the professional practice of CMHNs. First is a guiding paradigm, which involves respecting, valuing and facilitating the growth unique to each individual (Rogers 1990). Second, therapeutic presence is needed to restore clients' dignity and worth as healthy, unique human beings. Third, the therapeutic encounter, which is essential for healing and growth. Finally, the principles of CMHN, which include the search for recognised and unrecognised mental health needs; the prevention of a disequilibrium in mental health; the facilitation of mental health-enhancing activities; therapeutic approaches to mental health care and influences on policies affecting mental health (Long 2001).

Although several models are emerging in the organisation, delivery and evaluation of community mental health services, the guiding principles remain the same. Community profiling and collaborative working are considered by Long (2001) to be pivotal in promoting the mental health of the nation.

General practice nursing (GPN)

Nurses have been working in general practice for more than 80 years (Hyde 1995). Since the early 1990s, the number of practice nurses has grown considerably in response to the demands of general practice. The service expanded from 1515 nurses in 1982 to 10198 in 1998 (RCGP 2000). At the same time, the range of services they provide has also developed rapidly.

Practice nurses frequently fulfil the role of 'gatekeeper' and are relatively easily accessible and acceptable to patients as they are located within GP surgeries. The role of the practice nurse is wide-ranging and covers all age groups within the practice population (Saunders 2001). The types of service provided might include tasks such as ear syringing and venepuncture through to nurse-led chronic disease management programmes operated within agreed protocols. The expansion of nurse prescribing will enhance the provision of care for practice nurses working within clinics such as these (DOH 2000b). Chronic disease management and screening/secondary prevention programmes are areas of expertise for practice nurses, which could be further developed (Eve and Gerrish 2001). More recently, practice nurses have become involved in the implementation of NSF guidelines at a local level and often play a key role in establishing nurse-led clinics to tackle public health targets. For example, clinics for people with coronary heart disease.

School nursing

School nurses have been employed within the school health service for more than 100 years but have not been afforded, despite their importance, the same status as their community specialist practice colleagues, according to Thurtle (2001).

DeBell and Jackson (2000) state that the assessment of the specific health-care needs of school age children in the community is essential in the development of the school nursing service. They also emphasise that 'school nursing is committed to the health improvement of children and young people of school age'.

In addition to delivering core health surveillance programmes within schools, school nurses consider themselves to have particular responsibility for promoting healthy lifestyles and healthy schools; for child and adolescent mental health; chronic and complex health needs; and for vulnerable children and adolescents (Obeid 2001).

DOH (1999a, p.13) emphasises that school nurses are 'playing a vital role in equipping young people with the knowledge to make healthy lifestyle choices'. Key aspects of the school nurse's role include the assessment of health needs of children and school communities, agreement of individual and school plans and delivery of these through multi-disciplinary partnerships; playing a key role in immunisation and vaccination programmes; contributing to personal and health and social education and to citizenship training; working with parents to promote positive parenting; offering support and counselling, promoting positive mental health in young people and advising on and co-ordinating health care to children with medical needs.

In addition to this the DOH (1999b) identifies school nurses as public health practitioners with a specific role in the healthy school programme, tackling teenage pregnancy and working with families

Health visiting (HV)

The health visiting service has been in existence for more than 100 years and has its roots in public health and concern about poor health. The overall aim of the service is the promotion of health and the prevention of ill health. According to the Council for the Education and Training of Health Visitors (CETHV 1977), the four main elements of the health visitor's role are the search for health needs; stimulation of awareness of health needs; influence on policies affecting health; and facilitation of health-enhancing activities.

Although health visitors (HVs) will continue to maintain their public health role, they are also developing a much wider role in primary care. Traditionally, the focus of their work has been on monitoring the development of the under-fives. Several documents (Acheson 1998; DOH 1999a,1999b) have defined a new health agenda for the future, in which health visitors have a key role. A statement from *Making a Difference* (DOH 1999a, p. 132) reads: 'we are encouraging [health visitors] to develop a family-centred public health role, working with individuals, families and communities to improve health and tackle health inequality'. Family health maintenance, child protection and community outreach with vulnerable groups are examples of the type of work HVs undertake.

Appleby and Sayer (2001) stress the importance of health visitors finding new ways of measuring the effectiveness of their work, which tends to have long-term benefits for society but has always been notoriously difficult to quantify.

District nursing (DN)

District nurses can trace their roots back to the mid-1800s at least and the historical development of the service is well recorded. District nurses used to work in relative isolation but are more likely nowadays to work within a team (Thomas 2000). The role of the district nurse has evolved over time in response to political influences and the changing needs of the populations served. Although it is acknowledged that the role of the district nursing service is not clearly defined, it involves the assessment, organisation and delivery of care to support people living in their own homes (Audit Commission 1999). The three major elements of the role are that of clinical expert, manager and teacher (Clarridge *et al.* 2001). District nurses care for people with acute and chronic illnesses as well as those requiring palliative care. The majority of people on the district nurse's caseload tend to be from the older generation.

According to the RCN (2002a), the value of the district nursing service comes from its holistic approach to patient need and its ability to implement a package (often complex) of treatment that transcends health and social care. District nursing work is complex and wide ranging. Intermediate care, rehabilitation, rapid response and prevention of admission teams are current initiatives within the modernisation programme. District nurses are playing key roles in developing many of these innovative services.

Integrated nursing teams

Integrated nursing teams are 'teams of community-based nurses from different disciplines, working together within a primary care setting pooling their skills, knowledge and ability in order to provide the most effective care for their patients within a practice and the community it covers' (HVA 1996).

According to the Department of Health (1999a), integrated nursing teams are beneficial as they promote greater understanding of each other's roles, help to reduce duplication and allow for more targeted use of specialist skills.

Considering the acknowledged importance of tailoring services to patient need, an approach that responds to and addresses nursing/health issues identified as part of an individual or population-based health needs assessment exercise is preferable.

Example

A young child diagnosed with learning disabilities and who has associated physical health problems will require a comprehensive package of care. Working in alliance with a core integrated nursing team, which would include a health visitor, specialist services could be provided by a community children's nursing service and community learning disability nurses, ideally working in collaboration.

Beech (2002) explores the potential for integrated nursing teams in primary care settings and recognises that, at present, very little research-based evidence exists in relation to integrated nursing teams, particularly in terms of patient outcomes. She believes that all those people with a vested interest need to be consulted prior to the establishment of integrated teams and a structured approach is required for successful practice development.

GUARANTEEING A QUALITY SERVICE

With the launch of their new manifesto for health in 1997, the Labour government stressed the importance of delivering quality standards within the NHS:

> Professional and statutory bodies have a vital role in setting and promoting standards but shifting the focus towards quality will also require practitioners to accept responsibility for developing and maintaining standards within their local NHS organisations. For this reason, the Government will require every NHS Trust to embrace the concept of 'clinical governance' so that quality is at the core, both of their responsibilities as organisations and of each of their staff as individual professionals.
>
> (DOH 1997)

The DOH (1998b) reinforces the importance of ensuring that the services provided by health care professionals are of a high quality. The present government have established a number of organisations and initiatives designed to support a culture of excellence in health care: the National Institute for Clinical Excellence (NICE), national service frameworks (NSFs), the Commission for Healthcare Audit and Inspection (CHAI), the National Performance Framework, a National Survey of Patient and User Experience, and clinical governance (CG).

NICE provides advice on best practice with regard to existing treatments and evaluates new health interventions. In so doing, it encourages the use of the most appropriate treatments in terms of clinical and cost effectiveness.

NSFs are evidence-based national guidelines issued in relation to the treatment of specific client groups or disease categories. They act to ensure that people receive integrated, safe and clinically effective care (RCN 2002c). Collaborative practice is a prerequisite for the successful implementation of the NSFs. NSFs include strategies to support their implementation and establish performance milestones against which progress, within an agreed timescale, can be measured. NSFs form one of a number of initiatives designed to raise quality and decrease variations in service. There are plans to publish only one new framework annually. An external reference group (ERG) consisting of health professionals, service users and carers, health service managers, partner agencies and other advocates assists in the development of the NSFs with the support and supervision of the DOH. Since its launch in April 1998, the NSF programme has embraced established frameworks on cancer and paediatric intensive care and developed the mental health NSF (September 1999), the coronary heart disease NSF (March 2000), the national cancer plan (September 2000), the older person NSF (March 2001), the diabetes NSF (2001) and the children's NSF (2003). NSFs are being prepared for renal services and long-term neurological conditions.

The Commission for Healthcare Audit and Inspection (CHAI) is due to replace the Commission for Health Improvement (CHI), the national body that supports and monitors the quality of clinical governance and of clinical services. CHAI will be a more powerful health inspectorate, responsible for both public and private sectors. CHAI's other responsibilities will include conducting 'value for money' audits; determining star ratings for all NHS bodies and recommending special measures where necessary; validating performance assessment data, including waiting list information; reporting on NHS organisations' performance; providing independent scrutiny of patient complaints and reporting annually to parliament on health care progress and the resources that have been used. There are plans to create a single Commission for Social Care Inspection at the same time as CHAI, with a legal obligation on the two bodies to co-operate.

The National Performance Framework is designed to give a rounded picture of NHS performance and will address six areas: health improvement; fair access to services; effective delivery of appropriate healthcare; efficiency; patient/carer experience and health outcomes of NHS care.

The National Survey of Patient and User Experience is conducted annually to elicit the opinions of people in relation to care provided by the NHS.

The current government has proposed a 10-year modernisation programme for the NHS, which incorporates clear national standards, local delivery, statutory duty, life-long learning and professional self-regulation, monitoring of services through CHAI and the NHS Performance Framework and User survey. Clinical governance (CG) is the central concept that embraces all of these elements. It is a framework through which NHS organisations are accountable for continuously improving the quality of their services. According to Bennett and Robinson (2002), clinical governance is the vehicle for identifying not only excellence in care but also those aspects of practice that require further development.

The RCN (2002c) describes three main elements within clinical governance: quality improvement, risk management and management of performance and systems for accountability and responsibility. Quality improvement includes standard setting, clinical audit and evidence-based practice. Standards are devised in line with national/local clinical guidelines and evidence-based best practice and then implemented. Clinical audit is conducted to evaluate whether care meets the required standards and, where necessary, improvements are made, implemented and re-audited. Risk management involves all of those activities designed to promote best practice and avoid detrimental events happening. Individual practitioners are encouraged to view critical incidents and patient complaints positively and to learn from experiences, supported by a 'no blame' culture. In the clinical area, this involves clinical supervision, continuing professional development and effective clinical leadership. Within the wider NHS organisation, risk management systems might include incident reporting procedures and strategies/protocols to prevent adverse events. Systems for accountability and responsibility place a statutory responsibility for care within all NHS organisations. PCTs, and more specifically the chief executive, are responsible for the quality of care provided within their organisations. A clinician is appointed within each NHS organisation with responsibility for the implementation and evaluation of the CG framework. A spirit of teamworking and commitment to high standards of care is essential if CG is to be effective.

> ## Example
>
> In relation to your own organisation, consider ways in which the three elements of clinical governance – quality improvement, risk management and accountability, and responsibility – are implemented at a local level.

According to Zeh (2002), CG needs to be considered alongside professional self-regulation and continuing professional development. Increasingly, community specialist practitioners are being encouraged to develop their practice by discussing and sharing experiences with colleagues and regularly updating their skills, knowledge and expertise. In addition, there is a requirement to voice any concerns regarding compromised care and actively link into the wider organisational CG framework. Community nurses are accountable to the Nursing and Midwifery Council (NMC) and the public for the duties they perform. With CG, there are increased opportunities for patient involvement in decisions about care and more explicit mechanisms in place to make complaints and put forward their views.

FURTHER READING

Sines, D., Appleby, F. and Raymond, E. (eds) (2001) *Community Health Care Nursing* (2nd edn). Oxford: Blackwell Science.

Watson, N. and Wilkinson, C. (2001) *Nursing in Primary Care*. Basingstoke: Palgrave.

REFERENCES

Acheson, D. (1998) *Independent Inquiry into Inequalities in Health Report*. London: The Stationery Office.

Appleby, F. and Sayer, L. (2001) Public health nursing: health visiting. In D. Sines, F. Appleby and E. Raymond (eds), *Community Health Care Nursing*. Oxford: Blackwell Science.

Audit Commission (1993) *Children First: A Study of Hospital Services*. London: HMSO.

Audit Commission (1999) *First Assessment: A Review of District Nursing Services in England and Wales*. London: Audit Commission.

Barr, O. (2001) Community learning disability nursing. In D. Sines, F. Appleby and E. Raymond (eds), *Community Health Care Nursing*. Oxford: Blackwell Science.

Beech, M. (2002) The way forward? *Journal of Community Nursing*, 16(3): 46–8.

Bennett, J. and Robinson, A. (2002) Developing leadership capacity in community nursing: the context of change. *Journal of Community Nursing*,16(12): 4, 5.

Blaxter, M. (1990) *Health and Lifestyles*. London: Routledge.

Bollard, M. and Jukes, M.J.D. (1999) Specialist practitioners within community learning disability nursing and the primary health care team. *Journal of Learning Disabilities for Nursing, Health and Social Care*, 3(1): 11–19.

Bradshaw, J. (1972) The concept of social need. *New Society*, 30: 640–3.

Cain, P., Hyde, V. and Howkins, E. (1995) *Community Nursing: Dimensions and Dilemmas*. London: Arnold.

Council for the Education and Training of Health Visitors (1977) *An Investigation into the Principles of Health Visiting*. London: CETHV (reprinted 1993, London: ENB).

Chilton, S. and Barnes, E. (1997) Assessing health needs in the community. In S. Burley, E.E. Mitchell, K. Melling *et al.* (eds), *Contemporary Community Nursing*. London: Arnold.

Chorley, A. (2001) Occupational health nursing. In D. Sines, F. Appleby and E. Raymond (eds), *Community Health Care Nursing*. Oxford: Blackwell Science.

Clarke, J. (1999) Revisiting the concepts of community care and community health care nursing, *Nursing Standard*, 14(10): 34–6.

Clarridge, A., Boran, S. and Bninski, M. (2001) Contemporary issues in district nursing. In D. Sines, F. Appleby and E. Raymond (eds), *Community Health Care Nursing*. Oxford: Blackwell Science.

Cresswell, T. (1992) Assessing community health and social needs in North Derbyshire using participatory rapid appraisal. *Community Health Action*, 24.

Dahlgren, G. and Whitehead, M. (1991) *Policies and Strategies to Promote Social Equity in Health*. Stockholm: Institute for Future Studies.

DeBell, D. and Jackson, P. (2000) *School Nursing: A National Framework for Practice*. Consultation document. London: CPHVA.

Department of Health (1991) *The Welfare of Children and Young People in Hospital*. London: HMSO.

Department of Health/NHS Executive (1996) *Child Health in the Community: A Guide to Good Practice*. London: HMSO.

Department of Health (1997) *The New NHS: Modern, Dependable.* London: The Stationery Office.

Department of Health (1998a) *Our Healthier Nation: A Contract for Health.* Consultation document. London: The Stationery Office.

Department of Health (1998b) *A First Class Service: Quality in the New NHS.* London: The Stationery Office.

Department of Health (1999a) *Making a Difference: Strengthening the Nursing, Midwifery and Health Visiting Contribution to Health and Healthcare.* London: The Stationery Office.

Department of Health (1999b) *Saving Lives: Our Healthier Nation.* London: The Stationery Office.

Department of Health (2000a) *The NHS Plan: A Plan for Investment, A Plan for Reform.* London: The Stationery Office.

Department of Health (2000b) *Consultation on Proposals to Extend Nurse Prescribing.* London: The Stationery Office.

Department of Health (2001) *Shifting the Balance of Power within the NHS – Securing Delivery.* London: The Stationery Office.

Department of Health (2002) *Liberating the Talents: Helping Primary Care Trusts and Nurses to Deliver the NHS Plan.* London: The Stationery Office.

Department of Health and Social Security (1995) *Review of Policy for People with a Learning Disability.* Belfast: DHSS.

Eng, E., Salmon, M.E. and Mullan, I. (1992) Community empowerment: the critical base for primary health care. *Family and Community Health,* 15(1): 1–12.

Eve, R. and Gerrish, K. (2001) Roles, responsibilities and innovative capacity: the case of practice nurses. *Journal of Community Nursing,* 15(9): 4–6, 8.

Health Visitors' Association (1996) *Integrated Nursing Team: Initial Information.* Professional Briefing 1. London: HVA.

Hyde, V. (1995) Community nursing: a unified discipline? In P. Cain, V. Hyde and E. Howkins (eds), *Community Nursing: Dimensions and Dilemmas.* London: Arnold.

King's Fund (1994) *Community-oriented Primary Care.* London: King's Fund.

Latimer, J. and Ashburner, L. (1997) Primary care nursing: How can nurses influence its development? *Nursing Times Research,* 2(4): 258–67.

Long, A. (2001) Community mental health nursing. In D. Sines, F. Appleby and E. Raymond (eds), *Community Health Care Nursing.* Oxford: Blackwell Science.

Obeid, A. (2001) School health nursing review and recommendations for future practice. *Journal of Community Nursing,* 16(12): 6, 8, 10, 12, 15.

Quinney, D. and Pearson, M. (1996) *Different Worlds, Missed Opportunities: Primary Health Care Nursing in a North-western Health District.* Liverpool: Health and Community Care Research Unit, University of Liverpool.

Race, D.G. (1999) *Social Role Valorisation and the English Experience.* London: Whiting & Birch.

Rogers, C.R. (1990) *Client Centered Therapy.* London: Constable.

Royal College of General Practitioners (2000) *The Primary Care Workforce: An Update for the New Millennium.* London: RCGP.

Royal College of Nursing (1991) *A Guide to an Occupational Health Nursing Service: A Handbook for Employers and Nurses.* Middlesex: Scutari Projects Ltd.

Royal College of Nursing (2002a) *District Nursing: Changing and Challenging. A Framework for the 21st Century.* London: RCN.

Royal College of Nursing (2002b) *Community Children's Nursing. Information for primary care organisations, strategic health authorities and all professional working with children in community settings.* London: RCN.

Royal College of Nursing (2002c) *RCN Information: Guidance for Nurses on Clinical Governance.* London: RCN.

Saunders, M. (2001) General practice nursing. In D. Sines, F. Appleby and E. Raymond (eds), *Community Health Care Nursing.* Oxford: Blackwell Science.

Social Exclusion Unit (1999) *Teenage Pregnancy.* London: Social Exclusion Unit.

Thomas, S. (2000) The changing face of community nursing. *Primary Health Care,* 10(5): 21–4.

Thurtle, V. (2001) School nursing. In D. Sines, F. Appleby and E. Raymond (eds), *Community Health Care Nursing.* Oxford: Blackwell Science.

UK Central Council (1994) *Standards for Specialist Education and Practice.* London: UKCC.

Zeh, P. (2002) Clinical governance and the district nurse. *Journal of Community Nursing,* 16(4): 4, 6, 8, 11.

4

Personal safety in the community

Dee Drew

Learning outcomes

- Explain the importance of preparation needed prior to visiting patients and clients in their homes.
- Discuss considerations relating to personal safety when working in the community.
- Analyse interpersonal relationships in terms of non-confrontational behaviour.
- Discuss manual handling principles and their application to community settings.
- Clearly understand the importance of reporting incidents involving risk.

INTRODUCTION

Working in the community provides many challenges and opportunities. When placed in non-hospital settings as a student nurse or embarking upon a career as a community staff nurse, it is timely to reflect upon personal safety. This chapter is not intended to deter nurses from choosing to work in a community setting, but to ensure that practical and reasonable steps are taken to ensure their safety.

The first section of this chapter examines safety relating to the prevention and management of violence and aggression. The second part focuses upon manual handling, as the safety of both nurse and patient may be compromised if careful thought is not given to this issue before home visiting. The principles remain the same wherever the nurse is working, but some consideration needs to be made when moving into community settings. Finally, issues of reporting and bringing incidents to a resolution will be explored.

SAFETY AT WORK

The 1974 Health and Safety at Work Act and the 1992 Health and Safety at Work Regulations charge employers and employees with responsibilities in risky situations. Assessment of risk is a requirement to minimise potential harm and community nurses need to consider safety issues from both practical and professional perspectives.

Sadly, violence and aggression are an increasing problem in hospitals around the United Kingdom (Health Services Advisory Committee 1997, Royal College of Nursing 1998, Whittington and Wykes 1996). This is also the case for those nurses working in the community who are often working alone (Jackson, Clare and Mannix 2002) despite the Zero Tolerance Campaign launched in 1999 by the government.

This campaign sought to reduce the incidence of violence against nurses by 20 per cent. It has proved difficult to achieve (RCN 2001). It is very important to spend time considering how to prepare for community work and be aware of potential problems.

Exercise

Consider the differences between hospital working and being community-based. What health and safety issues may be encountered by community nurses?

BEING STREETWISE

This includes developing knowledge of the area of work, developing self-awareness and understanding why and how aggression can escalate.

First, learn the geography of the area, whether that is a town, clinic or surgery. Become familiar with the layout of rooms and buildings and note the position of exits. Find out what is known about the community. Without falling into the trap of stereotyping people, investigate what reputation the area has, find out about crime rates, for example. Talk to your colleagues about safety. It is strongly recommended (Leiba 1997) that visible security measures, involving personnel and technology, should be evident in health centres and clinics.

Exercise

The Ladybridge Estate is known to be a very deprived area with a high crime rate. Car theft and muggings are increasing.

List the precautions that could be taken by the community staff nurse prior to visiting a patient on the estate. Discuss your list with an experienced colleague/mentor.

There may be areas within the surrounding locality that are considered to be high risk. Sometimes community staff visit these in pairs. Find out if the remit of the post involves visiting after dark. It is good practice to gather as much information as is possible before setting off to a patient or client's house.

PREPARATION FOR HOME VISITING

This section will focus particularly upon home visits, as there are particular features that could,

potentially, compromise personal safety. Bearing this in mind, read carefully any records or notes pertaining to the visit. Talk to colleagues, who may know the situation and should make sure that concerns are shared. Look at the location of the visit – think about how you will get there.

Always remember that home visits, however welcome to the patient or client, are an invasion of that individual's space. Table 4.4 outlines some of the things that should be considered when arriving at someone's home.

The community nurse is a visitor in the patient's home and must wait to be invited in. It is good practice to discourage patients from leaving notes (for example: 'Please come round to the back – door open') and hanging keys on strings behind letterboxes. These, obviously, put patients at risk from unscrupulous opportunists. In addition to these measures, the community nurse should offer personal identification.

Compare the visits in the following example.

Example

Visit number 1

'Hello, I'm the nurse' (stepping over the threshold of the door). 'I'll just put my coat here and go and wash my hands.'

Visit number 2

'Hello, I'm Staff Nurse Winter from Greendale Health Centre' (showing her identification card). 'May I come in, Mrs Henry?' (enters on invitation). 'Is there somewhere that I could put my coat?' (waits for a reply). 'I need to wash my hands. Would it be OK to use your bathroom?'

The first visitor makes a number of assumptions. When a nurse gets to know the patient well, over a period of time, this kind of approach could be more acceptable, but remember that being in position of professional authority does not override common courtesy.

When visiting in other people's homes, self-

Table 4.1 *Entering a patient's home*

Considerations	Rationale
Remember that you are the visitor.	It is the patient's space that you are invading – it is unknown what is or has recently been happening in that person's home.
State clearly who you are and why you have come. Show your identity badge.	Don't assume that the person will recognise a uniform (if one is worn) or will be expecting the visit. It is good practice to encourage patients and clients to ask to see identification. This protects them as well as the professional.
Wait to be invited into the house and ask in which room the patient or client would like you to carry out the purpose for your visit.	Being pushy can make people irritated and angry. It may not be convenient for the patient or client to allow you into a particular room. This may be for good reason, e.g. if an unpredictable dog is shut in there!
Note the layout of the house – exits, telephones.	In case a speedy exit is required.
Be careful with people's property – protect their belongings.	Spillages, breakages or rough treatment of belongings will irritate – remember the visitor status.
Be alert – monitor moods and expressions during the visit.	Changes in the demeanour of the patient or client could indicate potential conflict developing.
Be self aware – monitor the manner in which information is given and care carried out. Do not react to conditions, which may seem unacceptable – dirty, smelly environments, for example.	The nurse should not provoke feelings of anger. Remember that this is the patient's home.
Trust instinctive feelings. If it feels that leaving quickly is the thing to do – go.	Often assessment of situations takes place on many levels. If uncomfortable feelings are building up don't wait until there is an incident.
If prevented from leaving – try not to panic – see the section relating to interpersonal relationships.	It may be possible for you to de-escalate the situation.

awareness is crucial. The conditions in which some people live can be upsetting. Monitoring facial expressions and choosing words carefully are a must (Leiba 1997). This may not prove to be easy. If so, take the opportunity to discuss your feelings with other members of the team after visits that leave emotions heightened.

The majority of home visits are very welcome to the patient or client. Relationships between community staff and the people that they care for can be very positive and a rewarding aspect of working in primary care. With thought, observation and self-awareness many potential problems may be avoided.

CAR SAFETY

Working in a community setting involves being mobile. In some localities bicycles may be an entirely appropriate way to get around; in busy cities public transport is often the best option. For most community staff, however, it would be impossible to function effectively without a car.

Some practical measures need to be undertaken relating to car safety (Table 4.2). Areas between car parks and clinic/surgery buildings should be well lit.

In addition to the above, it is helpful to plan the route to the destination with care. As the geography of the area becomes more familiar, this will become easier. Try not to give the impression that you are unsure of the way. Some police experts are now recommending that car doors are kept locked whilst driving in more dangerous areas. Good preparation for the journey makes it more likely that the nurse will arrive feeling calm. It is better to avoid road rage – especially if it is your own.

Walking between car and house, community nurses should appear purposeful, confident and in control. Walk towards the kerb side of the pavement and away from alleyways and hedges. Footwear should be comfortable and allow for speed, if necessary. It is not a good idea to wear jewellery at work for many reasons. Chains may catch or be pulled; rings and wristwatches are a hazard to patients and clients if physical care is needed. In addition to these (well known) considerations, wearing jewellery could catch the attention of muggers.

INTERPERSONAL RELATIONSHIPS AND NON-CONFRONTATIONAL BEHAVIOUR

In spite of the preparations suggested above, it may be that tensions rise whilst visiting. Confrontation may occur between patient or carer and nurse. Communication skills are crucially important in all fields of nursing; however, some issues need careful thought when visiting patients and clients in their own homes.

Households vary tremendously and staff new to community working may be surprised or shocked by the conditions in which some people live. An open mind needs to be cultivated in terms of the possible relationships that may be encountered – there are many variations of family life. It is necessary to communicate respect for all patients and clients, whatever thoughts may be experienced. Nabb (2000) found many incidences of family and carers assaulting nurses – remember that the giving and receiving of information should always be carried out courteously and sensitively.

Table 4.2 *Car safety*

Consideration	Rationale
It makes sense to ensure the vehicle is well maintained.	Not only is it inconvenient, it may be hazardous to break down in a remote place after dark. Well worth the expense of servicing and looking after the car.
Try not to run out of petrol.	The car will not be happy and again this could leave you stranded in remote or unsavoury places.
Park with thought.	Look for safe parking places. In the dark it is helpful to find a streetlight to park under. Try to park near to your destination.
Take out breakdown cover.	At least someone is coming to assist you. Always state that you are alone and make it clear if you are female.
Keep any nursing bags out of view – in addition to any personal valuables.	Some people may believe that nurses carry drugs in their bags – prevent temptation.

Table 4.3 *Interpersonal relationships – non-confrontational behaviour*

Considerations	Rationale
Be aware of how you are feeling and how you may appear to others.	If you appear worried or defensive you may cause worry or fear.
Try to look calm and relaxed.	Never try to domineer or act in an arrogant fashion. Attempts to belittle those who are angry are extremely dangerous.
Speak clearly and quietly – speak in a low pitch if possible.	Shouting or talking over others will provoke a response.
Listen to responses. Use non-verbal communication (such as nodding the head) to convey understanding.	This is a two-way process. Demands and commands should not be issued.
Try to accept how the other person is feeling. Ask for further clarification.	Even if the issue is difficult to empathise with, people own their feelings. Don't argue.
Be polite in the face of provocation.	Avoid becoming over-emotional. It is better to be brief and professional if tensions are mounting.
Try to ensure that the other person has an escape route.	If people are angry and feel crowded or cornered, aggression can be triggered.
Stay seated if the other person is seated.	It can be dangerous to tower over others – the aim is not to provoke.
Don't stand too close.	Leave reasonable personal space to avoid crowding.
Watch carefully to plan your exit.	Try to close the conversation if possible.

Table 4.3 suggests guidelines for non-confrontational behaviour to minimise the risk of provoking or encouraging aggression or violence. Some of the suggestions may appear to be 'common sense'. In situations of potential conflict, however, it is easy to feel anxious and behave inappropriately. Try to think carefully about the considerations and rationales before a difficult visit occurs.

Remember that there may be indicators that a person is potentially aggressive, such as using a raised voice, clenching their fists and threatening assault (Leiba 1997).

Exercise

Mr Grainger is very annoyed. David, the charge nurse, had told him that he would be visited on Tuesday. On Wednesday morning Mr Grainger rang the Health Centre to complain that no-one had been.

Consider the approach that should be taken when visiting Mr Grainger on Wednesday afternoon. Make notes of your decisions and discuss these with your team leader.

Aggression has been defined as:

> Any incident in which a health professional
> experiences abuse, threat, fear or the application
> of force arising out of the course of their work,
> whether or not they are on duty.

(RCN 1998: p.3)

This definition is useful, as actual abuse does not have to occur in order for aggression to be felt. Fear is a powerful enough experience to warrant action. The Royal College of Nursing's definition also does not differentiate between on- or off-duty situations. It is important to remember that insurance cover from employers relates to the duration of the shift.

ORGANISATIONAL SUPPORT

Under the 1974 Health and Safety at Work Act, employers have a duty to provide a safe working environment. Along with the responsibilities for employers there are also requirements, which need to be carried out by employees. Firstly, locate any policies and procedures, which exist locally relating to health and safety (RCN 1994). Study these carefully and note the reporting arrangements that are laid down for staff to follow.

Many primary care trusts (PCTs) offer training in assertiveness and dealing with aggression and violence. The Health and Safety at Work Regulations (1992) charge employers with provision of training in these fields. Take up the opportunities on offer. If there doesn't seem to be any training available ask if this could be arranged.

It is good practice to contact the work base at the end of the day to let someone know that visits are complete. The team leader will delegate visits to each member of staff and will co-ordinate the team. The order in which visits are carried out may not be predictable, but someone knows where each nurse should be visiting on a daily basis.

Many community nurses have the use of a mobile telephone, which can be useful in difficult situations. It may not be possible, however, to access the phone at the very time that you may need it. Mobile phones do not ensure safety, but they help. The use of personal alarms may be useful, to frighten, disorientate and debilitate an attacker. The Suzy Lamplugh Trust (see useful addresses) advises holding up the alarm directly to the ear of the attacker and running away as fast as possible.

In addition to all of the above, there is a potential threat (even in a 'caring profession'), which may not manifest itself in the homes or streets of the community served. Personal safety may be at risk in situations of harassment and bullying. Reported incidents are rising (Jackson, Clare and Mannix 2002; Rippon 2000) and it is important to be aware of ways to deal with bullies.

Bullying has been defined as the misuse of power or position (RCN 2001) and includes aggressive behaviour, ridiculing or humiliation, public criticism and exclusion from opportunities open to others.

Bullying may occur in any NHS setting and is, unfortunately, becoming more prevalent in many societies (Jackson, Clare and Mannix 2002). Many studies have found that aggression between staff is more upsetting and difficult to deal with than assaults from patients (Farrell 1999, 2001).

It is important not to keep bullying quiet – talk to other people (family, friends, trusted colleagues) and document what is happening. Employers are charged with the task of developing a culture of intolerance towards bullying and to deal with incidents effectively (DOH 2002). It is always better to try to address issues informally and directly at first – the person may not realise the effect that they are having. If, however, this does not work, then a formal complaint may be made. It is strongly advised that advice be sought from union representatives if a formal complaint is to be made.

A further requirement of the 1992 Health and Safety at Work Regulations is that of risk assessment in the workplace, which should be followed by planning, organising and monitoring both protective and preventive measures. The Health and Safety Executive (HSE) have issued a five-stage framework for risk assessment. This applies to all situations, which could lead to harm and is used also to evaluate needs relating to manual handling.

HSE'S FIVE STAGES OF RISK ASSESSMENT

These apply to all situations that have potential for risk. It is the case that many interventions carried out by nurses carry risks of harm to patients, the nurse and the general public. Dale and Woods (2001) state that these risks include clinical issues such as infection control, needlestick injury, inappropriate skill mix and staffing levels. There has been a rise in MRSA (methicillin-resistant *Staphylococcus aureus*) infections in community settings (Cookson 2000). This is of great concern and should mean that the highest standards are maintained in terms of hygiene.

Measures such as hand cleansing need to be carefully considered, particularly in patient's homes – not every household will have hot running water and soap, for example. Consult local policies for advice as to how to deal with this problem. There are many solutions for hand cleansing, in addition to traditional soap and water – these should be used as prescribed by the manufacturers. Uniforms and clothes worn for work need to be changed daily and laundered properly (RCN 1999b) to protect nurses and patients alike. Chronic understaffing puts nurses at risk. In addition to personal safety issues, health and safety within clinics and patient's homes needs consideration.

We shall now look at, each of the five stages of risk assessment and relate them to potentially threatening situations of violence or abuse.

1. Identify the hazards

This includes reports of threats and abuse, not only of actual physical violence, by patients, carers or others. Remember that this could be whether the nurse is on duty or not. The community staff nurse must report any incidents by following local policies.

Exercise

Select one of the identified hazards above. Locate local policies and procedures relating to that hazard and read them. Work through the stages of risk assessment with the chosen topic in mind. Discuss your thoughts with your team leader.

---

2. Identify who is at risk

Specify who could be harmed by the risk. This could include other members of the nursing team, other professionals and lay people.

3. Evaluate the risk

Assess the seriousness of the situation. Identify what can be done to minimise or eliminate the risk to protect those who could be harmed. Senior nurses will carry out the assessment of the risk with contributing evidence from the team. However, it is everyone's responsibility to identify and report potentially hazardous situations.

4. Record the findings

Decisions taken and workable measures to minimise the risk will be documented. This provides a working plan for staff and managers outlining all of the above in addition to steps, which may still need to be taken. Be sure to record events accurately (NMC 2002).

Poor communication of risk can result in misunderstanding and failure to pass on vital information to other colleagues. Documentation needs to be comprehensive and accurate, containing a full account of intervention and assessment of the situation (NMC 2002, Woods 2002). Avoid the use of jargon and abbreviations.

5. Review and revise the assessment

Assessment is a dynamic process. It is important to revisit the document, particularly after incidents are reported. Staff training and communications should also be reviewed.

It has been said that a major source of risk is uncertainty by members of staff about what is expected of them, especially in emergency situations (Dale and Woods 2001). Policies and procedures need to be current, available to those who need them, and comprehensive.

In order not to compromise patient care, care plans need to be regularly reviewed and updated so that staff are clear what has been found on assessment and what interventions are required.

The above stages also apply to other areas of practice – in the interests of patients and nurses it is important to think about manual handling situations arising in non-institutional settings.

MANUAL HANDLING IN THE COMMUNITY

The potential for safety to be compromised in manual handling situations in patients'/clients' homes is very real. The inclusion of this issue within this chapter is in recognition of the fact that over 30 per cent of nurses suffer work-related back pain each year (Institute of Employment Studies 1999).

Although the principles of manual handling remain the same wherever the nurse is working, community visiting gives rise to particular issues. By revisiting the five tenets of manual handling some of these are presented.

The task

There will be manual handling issues in many nursing procedures undertaken in the home (see Table 4. 4). These include moving patients in bed, helping patients get out of bed and standing up.

Toileting and dressing should be approached with thought, as should bathing and washing procedures.

The load

As in many settings, patients can be heavy and unpredictable. Paralysis, confusion or pain may make the patient a particular challenge.

When handling a load it is important to hold that load as close to the trunk as possible. Think about a patient in the middle of a double bed. This bed is low and not very firm. Immediately problems for safety (both for nurse(s) and patient) are apparent.

The environment

Nursing patients in their home environment is very different from doing so in a hospital ward. Hazards could include cluttered rooms with little space for manoeuvre, slippery polished floors, loose rugs and poor lighting. These are a problem for both patients and staff. It is important to address these hazardous conditions with tact and sensitivity. When rapport and trust have been developed between patient and nurse, suggestions for improving home safety will be better received.

The worker

Nurses come in all shapes and sizes. The same is true of carers, who tend to be more involved in giving direct care in home settings. Older people

---

Table 4.4 *Occasions when manual handling procedures must be carefully considered*

1   *Moving patients in bed*

2   *Helping them to sit or stand up*

3   *Toileting and dressing*

Note the following:

A full assessment will be carried out as required according to the Manual Handling Operations Regulations 1992.

The sister or charge nurse will assess patients. Measures to reduce the risk of potential injury will be put in place, e.g. a hospital bed may need to be provided.

The assessment will be documented in the care plan. Any changes in circumstances must be reported to the team leader.

who are carers may not be in the best of health themselves. It is important not to make assumptions about the abilities of others.

The organisation

Policies and procedures relating to manual handling must be studied carefully (Chambers 1998). Mandatory updates in PCTs are necessary to ensure the safety of staff and patients. There may be unfamiliar equipment in patients' homes. Don't use unknown manual handling aids until training has been carried out.

Inadequate staffing levels can put nurses at risk. The number of staff at any given time will affect directly the workload of each nurse. Tired staff are more vulnerable to injuries, accidents and mistakes (RCN 1996, 1999a).

In addition to the above, keeping fit and healthy can reduce the possibility of back problems developing. By valuing and safeguarding his/her own health the community nurse can contribute to the risk reduction process.

REPORTING INCIDENTS

Nurses are required to report issues relating to safety under the Health and Safety at work Act (1974). If injury occurs as a result of manual handling procedures, then this must be reported.

There is evidence that a large majority of nurses believe that a certain level of aggression is part of the job (Leiba 1997, Unison 1997). This acceptance of abuse seems to be particularly widespread amongst older nurses. In their campaign to 'stamp out violence', the *Nursing Times* received 1000 replies to a questionnaire on the subject (Coombes 1998). In nurses aged over 55 years, 92 per cent felt that violence and aggression was part of the nurse's lot. Amongst nurses aged between 26 and 34 this view was held by 76 per cent. Undoubtedly this leads to an underreporting of incidents, which is worrying. It will not be possible to gauge the size of the problem if nurses are reluctant to speak up. It is also unfair to colleagues to keep quiet. Today might have included verbal abuse from a relative, tomorrow (particularly if the situation is poorly handled) may lead to something much worse.

The report should be made as soon as is possible. Events should be clearly and comprehensively stated.

Exercise

Find out the procedure for reporting incidents of abuse within your primary care team. Who could be helpful in these situations? Locate the Occupational Health Department and explore the services offered by its staff.

SUPPORT AND COUNSELLING

People who have been involved in aggressive or violent incidents need to be supported at work. Reporting the events can be traumatic and it is helpful to have assistance from a colleague when completing the necessary documentation (RCN 1998). It may be helpful to discuss what has happened with other members of staff. A debriefing should take place with the people concerned. The actual events should be explored, including any possible triggering factors and the feelings of those who took part. Ways of preventing recurrence should be considered.

Commonly, following verbal abuse or physical attack feelings of fear, guilt or anger may be experienced. These can manifest themselves in taking the 'blame' for provoking aggression, wondering if the experience will be repeated or anger towards the aggressor, the organisation or even oneself.

It may take time for a victim of abuse or violence to regain the confidence to visit alone again. Support may be offered by occupational health, professional organisations or counselling services. Support may also be needed for others involved, including the aggressor.

CONCLUSION

After careful consideration of the issues addressed within this chapter, turn back to the learning outcomes at the beginning and think about each one in turn. Look back at the notes made for the first exercise at the beginning of this chapter. Is there anything that you would like to add to them?

If this chapter has raised any concerns for practice, it is important that they are discussed with an experienced community nurse, either informally or through clinical supervision channels. Some useful addresses can be found at the end of this section.

Remember that the majority of staff working in community settings enjoy a close partnership with their patients and clients. The health centre or surgery is at the heart of the local community and relationships may build over a number of years. Visiting patients and clients in their homes is a privilege that greatly enhances the experience of community nursing. Taking practical precautions and taking time to think about safety can better prepare the community nurse for difficult situations that could arise.

FURTHER READING

Anderson, L.N. and Clarke, J.T. (1996) De-escalating verbal aggression in primary care settings. *Nurse Practitioner American Journal of Primary Health Care*, 21(10): 95.

RCN (2002) *Code of Practice for Patient Handling*. London: Royal College of Nursing.

REFERENCES

Chambers, N. (1998) The experience of being the registered nurse on duty: managing a violent incident involving an elderly patient. *Journal of Advanced Nursing*, 2: 429–36.

Cookson, B. (2000) Methicillin-resistant *Staphylococcus aureus* in the community – new battlefronts or are the battles lost? *Infection Control Hospital Epidemiology*, 21(6): 398–403.

Coombes, R. (1998) Violence, the facts. *Nursing Times*, 94(43): 12–14.

Dale, C. and Woods, P. (2001) A risk assessment and management strategy for community nursing. *British Journal of Community Nursing*, 5(6): 286–91.

Department of Health (2002) *Improving Working Lives*. London: DOH. www.doh.gov.uk/iw/index.htm

Farrell, G.A. (1999) Aggression in clinical settings – a follow-up study. *Journal of Advanced Nursing*, 29: 532–41.

Farrell, G.A. (2001) From tall poppies to squashed weeds: why don't nurses pull together more? *Journal of Advanced Nursing* 35(1): 26–33.

Health and Safety at Work Act (1974). London: HMSO.

Health and Safety at Work Regulations (1992). London: HMSO.

Health Services Advisory Committee (1997) *Violence and Aggression to Staff in Health Services*. Sheffield: HSE Books.

Institute of Employment Studies (1999) Royal College of Nursing. Unpublished data from RCN membership survey.

Jackson, D., Clare, J. and Mannix, J. (2002) Who would want to be a nurse? Violence in the workplace – a factor in recruitment and retention. *Journal of Nursing Management* 10(1): 13–23.

Leiba, T. (1997) Tackling aggression and violence in the workplace. *Managing Clinical Nursing*, 129–34.

Nabb, D. (2000) Visitors' violence: the serious effects of aggression on nurses and others. *Nursing Standard*, 14: 36–8.

Nursing and Midwifery Council (2002) *Guidelines for Records and Record keeping*. London: NMC.

Rippon, T. (2000) Aggression and violence in health care professions. *Journal of Advanced Nursing* 31(2): 452–60.

Royal College of Nursing (1994) *Violence and Community Staff – Advice for Managers*. London: RCN.

Royal College of Nursing (1996) *Manual Handling Assessments in Hospital and the Community*. London: RCN.

Royal College of Nursing (1998) *Dealing with Violence against Nursing Staff*. London: RCN.

Royal College of Nursing (1999a) *Changing Practice – Improving Health: An Integrated Back Injury Prevention Programme for Nursing and Care Homes*. London: RCN.

Royal College of Nursing (1999b) *Taking a Uniform Approach: An RCN Guide to Selecting the Right Clothing for Nurses*. London: RCN.

Royal College of Nursing (2001) *Working Well: A Call to Employers. A Summary of the RCN's Working Well Survey into the Well-being and Working Lives of Nurses*. London: RCN.

Unison (1997) *Violence at Work: Health Staff Survey*. London: Unison.

Whittington, R. and Wykes, T. (1996) An evaluation of staff training in psychological techniques for the management of patient aggression. *Journal of Clinical Nursing*, 5: 257–61.

Woods, C. (2002) The importance of good record-keeping for nurses. *Nursing Times*, 99(2): 26–7.

USEFUL CONTACTS

Victim Support
Cranmer House
39 Brixton Road
London
SW9 6DZ
Tel. 0171 7359166

Victim Support
14 Frederick Street
Edinburgh
EH2 2HB
Tel. 0131 2258233

The Suzy Lamplugh Trust
14 East Sheen Avenue
London
SW14 8AS
Tel. 020 83921839

Royal College of Nursing Counselling Service
Tel. 0345 697064

www.freedomtonurse.co.uk
Freedom to Nurse
P.O. Box 37
Worksop
Nottingham
S80 1ZT

5

Therapeutic relationships

Patricia Wilson and Sue Miller

Learning outcomes

- Identify the features of a therapeutic relationship.
- Discuss some of the challenges for community nurses in establishing a therapeutic relationship.
- Recognise some of the issues that may arise when trying to establish a therapeutic relationship with specific patients.
- Explore some of the possible consequences of failing to establish a therapeutic relationship.
- Analyse the impact of changes in policy on the development of therapeutic relationships.

This chapter will focus upon the relationship that exists between the nurse, patient and their family. It is recognised that such a relationship should be therapeutic, and indeed this would seem essential to the delivery of effective nursing care. However, it is unwise to assume a therapeutic relationship will automatically occur, as there are many challenges in establishing and maintaining such a relationship in community settings. In this chapter the key features of a therapeutic relationship will be identified and some of the challenges of maintaining that relationship in a community setting will be discussed. This will lead the reader to consider some of the issues of particular relevance to her patient group, and to explore some of the consequences of failing to establish and maintain relationships. In conclusion, the current and potential changes in health care delivery will be reviewed with particular reference to the way these changes might impact on the nurse/patient/family relationship.

THE FEATURES OF A THERAPEUTIC RELATIONSHIP

The recognition of the importance of the therapeutic relationship is not a new phenomenon.

Peplau's (1952) theory of nursing is based upon the importance of the relationship between the nurse and the patient, and she asserts this is the way in which all nursing care is delivered. The importance of this relationship has continued to be widely acknowledged and indeed McMahon and Pearson (1998) suggest that it is central to patient health, well-being and recovery. Since a therapeutic relationship is so important, it is essential to consider what features characterise such a relationship. In reviewing various definitions it becomes apparent that the important factors are:

- appropriate boundaries are maintained
- meets the needs of the patient
- promotes patient autonomy
- positive experience for the patient.

Appropriate boundaries are maintained

A boundary, as defined in the dictionary (Chamber, 1993) is: 'a limit, a border, termination or final limit'. Within the therapeutic relationship, boundaries define how far the nurse is willing to go to meet the needs of the patient and his family.

Therefore it is important that the nurse, patient and family are clear regarding their relationship and what is reasonably expected of each party. This will protect all those involved in the relationship. A publication from the UK Central Council (1999: p.5) on this subject states that: 'boundaries define the limits of behaviour which allow a client and practitioner to engage safely in a therapeutic, caring relationship'. The practitioner has the responsibility to maintain appropriate professional boundaries at all times (UKCC 1999). However, the process of finding the boundaries of care is far from automatic (Totka 1996), as will be discussed later in this chapter.

Meets the needs of the patient

The purpose of the relationship between the nurse and patient is to meet the nursing needs of that patient. It is therefore important that the nursing needs of the patient are discussed at the outset of the relationship in order that mutually identified goals can be set and each person within the relationship can be clear as to their role in the achievement of those goals. This might include the nurse, patient, family members, other professionals and carers. This will require expert communication skills on the part of the nurse in order that a relationship of trust can develop. Whilst the relationship exists to meet the needs of the patient it is likely that the nurse will experience satisfaction in helping the patient to meet those needs. This is entirely appropriate. However, it is important that nurses do not allow their personal needs for positive self-esteem, control and belonging to undermine the professional relationship (Jerome and Ferraro-McDuffie 1992). This requires the nurse to be self-aware and open to seeking support from others when the need arises.

Promotes patient autonomy

Autonomy is the right to self-determination. Self-determination can be defined as an ability to understand one's own situation, to make plans and choices and to pursue personal goals (McParland *et al.* 2000). This further supports the need for excellent communication skills on the part of the nurse in order to assist the patient to understand

their own situation. Within a relationship that promotes patient autonomy the patient will contribute to the achievement of personal goals and will move towards independence.

Positive experience for the patient

The experience of participating in a therapeutic relationship will be positive for the patient as nursing needs will be met, in a way that is most appropriate to the patient and their family. Truly therapeutic relationships can empower the patient, the family and the nurse.

These features are embodied in the Code of Professional Conduct, which states:

> You must at all times, maintain appropriate professional boundaries in the relationships you have with patients and clients. You must ensure that all aspects of the relationship focus exclusively upon the needs of the patient or client.

(NMC 2002: Clause 2.3)

Exercise

Think about entering a patient's home and establishing a therapeutic relationship. What skills do you have that would enable you to achieve this? What skills need further development? How can you develop your skills further? Discuss your ideas with your mentor/preceptor.

CHALLENGES OF DEVELOPING THERAPEUTIC RELATIONSHIPS IN COMMUNITY SETTINGS

Having considered the features of a professional relationship, some of the challenges of achieving such a relationship in the community setting will be discussed. Professional relationships with the patient are influenced by a number of factors – illustrated in Figure 5.1.

Location of care

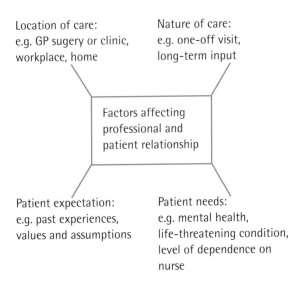

Location of care:
e.g. GP sugery or clinic,
workplace, home

Nature of care:
e.g. one-off visit,
long-term input

Factors affecting
professional and
patient relationship

Patient expectation:
e.g. past experiences,
values and assumptions

Patient needs:
e.g. mental health,
life-threatening condition,
level of dependence on
nurse

Figure 5.1 *Factors affecting the therapeutic relationship*

The delivery of care within the home can provide a feeling of security for the patient and his carer/s as they are on familiar territory. This can make it easier to develop a good relationship, such that they are able to share their concerns and worries. It is also probable that patients and carers will be able to learn new skills more readily as they are likely to feel more relaxed within their 'normal' environment.

In this example the benefits of home visiting are apparent. These opportunities could be lost if health visitors change their mode of practice to give more care in clinic settings, as has been reported by Normandale (2001). However, caring in the home environment can leave the nurse feeling vulnerable. A nurse who has recently left a hospital-based job to work in the community can feel very isolated. Despite the use of mobile phones and pagers it is more difficult to seek the advice of a colleague, and help may not be instantly at hand. A nurse who feels vulnerable and isolated will find it more difficult to inspire the confidence of patients.

Working in the relative isolation of the home can provide challenges to nurses in maintaining standards of care. If the relationship is not 'therapeutic' it can be difficult for the nurse to identify this herself, particularly if the situation has developed over time. The support and guidance of colleagues is essential, as is the willingness of the nurse to be open to that support. Totka (1996) notes that peers often recognise unhealthy situations before the nurse involved, but find it difficult to discuss the situation with their colleague.

Care given by the nurse within the workplace will also be different from the more traditional hospital setting. The occupational health nurse works within a three-way relationship between the employer, employee and the nurse (Atwell 1996).

Example

Consider Mrs Patel, whose 2-year-old son has recently been in hospital suffering from an asthmatic attack. Mrs Patel speaks some English but found the experience of her son being in hospital very stressful. When the health visitor made a visit to the home Mrs Patel was unsure how to use the prescribed medication, particularly the use of the spacer device to administer the inhalers. Teaching Mrs Patel at home is likely to be more successful, as she will be more relaxed and it will be possible for the health visitor to reinforce any aspects of the care at a later date if this is necessary.

Example

Although stress in the workplace is being increasingly recognised as a legitimate occupational health issue (Health and Safety Executive 2000), many employees will still consider it unwise for their career prospects to report mental health needs to their occupational health nurse. The challenge for the nurse within this context is to promote trust with the employees in order to facilitate a therapeutic relationship.

Developing therapeutic relationships may also be affected by a clinic or surgery setting, where the patient may gain the impression of busy workloads inhibiting the time they spend with the nurse. Paterson (2001) identified lack of time as a major inhibitor in developing a participatory relationship between professional and patient, and although the nurse is likely to be as busy, if not more so, when undertaking home visits the interaction may be less distracted than in a busy clinic.

Example

Consider the scenario of the new mother trying to explain her depression to the health visitor and how much harder this might be in a busy baby clinic rather than in the privacy of her own home.

In other cases the relative anonymity the surgery or clinic provides may be of benefit in facilitating the development of a therapeutic relationship. Initial assessments are often the first point of contact between community nurse and patient and the nurse must develop skills to enable a conducive environment in order to establish the start of a therapeutic relationship (Bryans and McIntosh 1996).

Exercise

Do you wear a uniform when working in the community? What are the advantages and disadvantages of wearing a uniform? If you had a choice would you wear a uniform?

Working in the community, many nurses find that not wearing a uniform removes an unnecessary barrier, which makes the development of a therapeutic relationship an easier task. It does, however, require skills on the part of the nurse to gain access to the patient's home, gain the patient's trust and explain her nursing role, since a symbol, which for many carries some degree of status, has been lost.

For those community nurses who do wear a uniform other challenges arise. Wearing of a

uniform can enable almost instant entry to some homes, but may present a barrier to acceptance by some people. This may be especially apparent with children, who have perhaps learnt to associate uniforms with pain and discomfort. In these situations it will take time to address prior conceptions before a therapeutic relationship can be established.

If nurses do not wear a recognised uniform it is particularly important to consider the appropriateness of the clothing that is worn. Entering a home inappropriately dressed may cause offence and prevent establishment of a relationship. Perhaps this might require the nurse to cover her arms and legs if visiting Asian families, or maybe to remove shoes prior to entry into some homes. In order to meet the needs of individual families the nurse must enquire as to family preferences and be willing to adapt behaviours to respect values different from her own, in order to facilitate good relationships.

A final point about dress code: whether wearing uniform or not, it is essential to carry identification at all times in order to protect the wellbeing of patients.

Nature of care

Exercise

Have you cared for a patient over a long period of time? How did your relationship with the patient develop? Did you find yourself becoming 'closer' to the patient? How did this make you feel? Discuss this with your mentor/preceptor.

A key element in the nature of the therapeutic relationship with all patient groups is the duration of the relationship. Morse (1991) describes three appropriate relationships. Firstly, she describes the one-off clinical encounter that, for example, a practice nurse may have with a patient in a travel clinic. There are also encounters that last longer but focus on a specific need, such as maintenance of hormone replacement therapy. Both of these relationships are mutual and appropriate to certain situations but Morse argues that within a much longer-term nurse–patient relationship there should be a different focus, with the development of what Morse terms as a connected relationship. Morse suggests that the key characteristic of a connected relationship is that the nurse views the patient as a person first rather than a patient.

Example

A district nurse has been visiting an elderly lady for several years. The visits now may often include a chat over a cup of tea about how the grandchildren are progressing or other issues in the patient's life on which the nurse has developed a wealth of knowledge over the years. Although it may be a venous ulcer that initiated the referral to the district nurse, the connected relationship that has developed with time allows the nurse to deal with other issues that may be far more important to the patient, such as feelings of loneliness. During the chat a skilled nurse will be able to assess for signs of depression or other psychosocial needs that are common in chronic illness.

Whilst for many families and professionals this can only be positive, there is a potential to step over the professional boundary and it is essential to maintain the appropriate balance within the therapeutic relationship. The consequences of not maintaining the balance will be explored later in the chapter.

Exercise

Have you ever cared for a patient who did not follow the recommended treatment programme? Why did the patient not adhere to the treatment regimen? How did it make you feel?

In the home environment the patient and his carer could be perceived to have greater control within the relationship. Should the patient decide not to concur with recommended treatment, this may not be immediately evident as the nurse is spending only a short period of time within the home environment. Parkin (2001) notes that professionals are unable to control the home environment. If, unbeknown to the nurse, the patient has not adhered to the recommended treatment, the therapeutic relationship is threatened, since a relationship based on trust no longer exists. Within a therapeutic relationship the patient should be able to tell the nurse of his intentions. This might allow treatment to be modified such that the patient feels able to follow the regimen, but even if this is not the case at least the nurse is aware of the true situation and can modify her nursing care accordingly.

Example

Susie is 14 years old and has been diabetic for 3 years. She is supposed to record her blood glucose levels once daily, varying the time of day she takes the readings, but she finds this requirement tiresome and does not do it. Prior to the community children's nurse's visit she wonders what to do – should she make up some values to keep the nurse happy or should she tell the truth? Hopefully if Susie and the nurse have a good relationship she can be truthful and they can work together on what care Susie can reasonably be expected to give herself.

Further exploration of the current and future context of concordance can be found in the last section of this chapter.

Patient expectations

Expectations of the nurse and of the community nursing service may also impact on the relationship between the nurse and adult patient. Over the past 25 years there has been a rapid rise in consumerism (May and Purkis 1997), with a corresponding rise in expectations of the Health Service. In community nursing this can be seen by the use of time bands in allocating home visits and the proliferation of charters and mission statements displayed on clinic and surgery walls.

Many patients have clear ideas on the service they expect from community nurses with a consequential detrimental effect on the therapeutic relationship when these expectations are either not met or are unrealistic.

However, despite trends in healthy ageing and participation in health care (Lorig *et al.* 1996), many older adults were bought up in a society where medicine was seen to have all the answers and the public was expected to be the passive recipient of care (Dukes Hess 1996). There is some evidence that not all adult patients wish to be an active partner in the therapeutic relationship (Waterworth and Luker 1990) and there may be a significant number of patients who feel more comfortable with the paternalistic model of care (Roberts 2001). The nurse 'doing for' the patient rather than enabling them to self-care contradicts the current trend towards empowerment (Copperman and Morrison 1995), which is a central theme in the *National Service Framework for Older People* (DOH 2001a). The community nurse may find a challenge in helping some patients in developing the confidence and ability to self care, and again the therapeutic relationship will be focused on trust and the facilitation of realistic independence.

Patient needs

The main purpose of the nursing or health visiting intervention may also have a significant impact on the therapeutic relationship. The patient within the relationship may have significant physical and emotional needs, such as happens in palliative care. The relationship in such cases may be based on intensive input by the nurse (Goodman *et al.*1998). In contrast, the practice nurse or occupational health nurse may see a person for health screening with less obvious health needs as the focus of the intervention.

The substantial shift of care from hospitals to the community for those with mental health needs (Brooker and Repper 1998) has resulted in a rapidly developing role for community nurses in supporting this group. With approximately one in six people at any one time suffering from mental illness in the United Kingdom (DOH 1999a) the role is constantly evolving. *The National Service Framework for Mental Health* (DOH 1999a) is firmly underpinned by a patient focus. However, empowering patients with mental health needs is often challenging, not least because of concerns from society and professionals as to whether some patients have the capability of making decisions over their care and treatment (Feenan 1997).

Table 5.1 *Responses to caring role*

Response to caring role	Features of response
Engulfment mode	<ul><li>*Cannot articulate needs as a carer*</li><li>*No other occupation*</li><li>*Generally female spouse*</li><li>*Total sense of responsibility and duty*</li></ul>
The balancing/boundary setting mode	<ul><li>*Have a clear picture of themselves as carers (e.g. how they save nation money)*</li><li>*Generally male*</li><li>*Often adopt language of an occupation – treat role as a job*</li><li>*May emotionally detach themselves from recipient*</li></ul>
Symbiotic mode	<ul><li>*Positive gain by caring*</li><li>*Does not want role taken away*</li></ul>

Adapted from Twigg and Atkin (1994)

The therapeutic relationship with this group is essential in empowering patients to actively participate in decisions about their care. Peplau's (1952) developmental model is often used as the framework for developing a therapeutic relationship (Collister 1986) with the assessment (or orientation) phase focusing on the development of mutual trust and regard between nurse and patient, as well as data gathering. Addressing anxiety is the overarching aim of the therapeutic relationship (Aggleton and Chalmers 2000), and the community nurse may take on a number of roles to facilitate this including that of counsellor, resource, teacher, leader or surrogate. All nurses working in the community develop knowledge of local resources and other agencies and facilitating the patient to access these may be the key component within this relationship.

It should also be acknowledged that the therapeutic relationship in the community setting is not only formed between nurse and patient, but will often encompass an informal carer. In the United Kingdom there are approximately 6 million informal carers who are the primary carers for a range of patients ranging from young people with learning disabilities, to the frail elderly (Bond *et al.* 1999). The Carers Recognition and Services Act (DOH 1995) and the Carers and Disabled Childrens Act (DOH 2000) enshrined the principle that carers should be assessed and acknowledged as an individual rather than simply an adjunct to the patient. For the community nurse this reinforces that an individual therapeutic relationship must also be developed with the informal carer, but this poses a number of challenges.

First, a significant number of informal carers are unknown to the community nurse, with Henwood (1998) estimating that only half of all carers receive any support from community nurses. Second, the more an informal carer does for the patient, the less intervention there will be from the community nurse (Pickard *et al.* 2000). Consequently, the informal carers most likely to benefit from a therapeutic relationship are less likely to be visited by the community nurse. Third, there are often misguided assumptions by many professionals that informal carers should undertake the caring role and that the role is taken on very willingly (Procter *et al.* 2001).

Finally, studies have shown that many informal carers have significant health needs of their own which often are unrecognised (Henwood 1998) and undertake very complex and technical tasks (Pickard *et al.* 2000). All too frequently community nurses first meet an informal carer when there is a crisis and the nursing input is a short-term measure to help the patient and carer over this period. However, the therapeutic relationship with informal carers should ideally be long-term, with the nurse aiming to provide information and acting as a resource (Seddon and Robinson 2001) and responding to the role the carer is happy to undertake.

Twigg and Atkin (1994) describe three different responses by individuals to the informal caring role, given in Table 5.1.

It is important for the community nurse to recognise the informal carer's response to their situation.

Example

Imagine the case of Lily, a 75-year-old mother caring for her son Ted, who has Down's syndrome. She is devoted to her son and has no other life than caring for him. The General Practitioner has referred Ted for a wound assessment but when the nurse arrives it is apparent that Lily is exhausted by her role. The challenge for the nurse is to establish a relationship that enables Lily to acknowledge her individual needs and helps her to accept help without feelings of guilt. This may involve developing a long-term relationship and not simply the organising of respite, which many informal carers do not want (Pickard *et al.* 2000).

Another frequently met scenario is that of the husband caring for his wife. He has every detail organised and is business-like in his approach to the community nurse. Again, this may hide a number of physical and emotional needs, and the community nurse must develop a therapeutic relationship in order to enable him to express these. The needs of informal carers are only now being recognised and the community nurse must develop a relationship and provide intervention appropriate to both the patient and informal carer as individuals.

WHEN THE BALANCE IS NOT MAINTAINED: FAILURES IN THERAPEUTIC RELATIONSHIPS

Exercise

How do you define friendships? Have you ever been in a situation when a patient wanted to be your friend? What would you do if a patient wanted to develop a friendship with you? Discuss your ideas with a professional colleague.

In reality it is hard to learn about boundaries unless one is involved in setting them, and extending beyond the therapeutic boundary may only be apparent once it has been breached.

Example

Consider the case of Ann who is John's community children's nurse. Ann has cared for John, aged 5, for the last 2 years and supported Gill, his single mother, through some difficult times, as John has received treatment for acute lymphoblastic leukaemia. During Ann's recent visit to the home Gill and John invite her to John's 6th birthday party the following weekend. Ann considers this briefly and agrees to come. At the end of the party Gill asks Ann if she would be willing to baby-sit for John, as she's the only person she feels she can trust to care for John. What should she do now? It would appear the edges of the professional boundary have become significantly blurred such that Gill feels it is appropriate to ask Ann to baby-sit.

It may be that it is in the interests of the patient and his carer to encourage the professional to develop a relationship of friendship since this has the potential to 'normalise' the patient, as it is 'normal' to have friends who visit. This is perhaps more likely to occur if nurses do not wear uniforms. Families may be keen that friendships do develop since a friend is likely to respond to requests for help, perhaps more swiftly than a detached professional. Therefore nurses must consider their actions carefully in case actions are misinterpreted, as perhaps was the case when Ann attended John's party.

Hylton Rushton et al. (1996) describes over-involvement as a lack of separation between the nurse's own feelings and that of the patient. Typically the nurse may spend off-duty time with the patient (Barnsteiner and Gillis-Donovan 1990), appear territorial over the care (Morse 1991), or treat certain patients with favouritism (Wilson 2001a). Consequences for the patient are an over-dependence on that particular nurse and a lack of support in reaching therapeutic goals. For the community nurse the implications are often significant stress and deterioration in job satisfaction (Hylton Rushton et al. 1996) and an inevitable detrimental effect on team working.

Of course, the balance in the therapeutic relationship may be tipped the other way. The detached, cold nurse who seems indifferent to her patient's emotional needs may be familiar to the reader. The results of under-involvement are a lack of understanding by the nurse of the patient's perspective, conflict, and standardised rather than contextually dependant care (Hylton Rushton et al. 1996). It has been suggested that the overwhelming feelings that a nurse may have for a patient's situation can lead to dissociation by the nurse within the therapeutic relationship (Crowe 2000). Within the community setting the feelings of being the last resort in care has also been linked to under-involvement within the therapeutic relationship (Wilson 2001a). The consequences of under-involvement for the patient is that the nurse has a lack of insight into the patient's perspective and is unable to facilitate the patient in meeting therapeutic goals.

Exercise

Think of a likeable patient who you have recently cared for. Reflect on the following: What were the characteristics of this patient and their care that made it a positive experience for you? If other colleagues were involved do you think they felt the same way? Was the care you gave this patient affected by these feelings? Are there any consequences for yourself, the patient, your other patients?

Maintaining a therapeutic relationship is particularly challenging in the community nursing context because of the commonly intense nature of care, duration of contact and the non-clinical environment. Reflection with colleagues and clinical supervision become invaluable tools to facilitate the nurse in developing the appropriate relationship with patients.

THE INFLUENCE OF THE CURRENT AND FUTURE CONTEXT ON THERAPEUTIC RELATIONSHIPS

Long-term interventions within the community setting will continue to increase with an ageing population and rise in chronic illness (Kalache 1996; Wellard 1998; DOH 1999b), and this chapter has already explored the impact of duration of care on the therapeutic relationship. One response by policy makers to the rise in long-term conditions is the facilitation of individuals to self-manage their own conditions. The expert patient programme (DOH 2001b) recognises that individuals often have significant expertise about their chronic illness which has developed over years through experience and the aim of the programme is to further develop this expertise in order to promote symptom control, quality of life and effective use of health resources (Wilson 2001b). Within all spheres of community nursing, nurses are now dealing with far more knowledgeable patients not least because of the readily available access to information via the Internet (Timmons 2001). Therapeutic relationships in the current climate must be based on an acknowledgement that the patient may have considerable expertise in their own condition, exceeding that of the nurse. There has been some debate as to how comfortable community nurses are with this (Wilson 2002), but there can be little doubt that a therapeutic relationship that fails to take into account the knowledge that both nurse and patient bring will fail.

The expert patient programme is one example of a policy that is based on partnership and responsibility (Wilson 2001b). Another example is the move towards concordance (Royal Pharmaceutical Society of Great Britain 1997), where the patient's views are considered of equal importance in treatment plans.

> ### Exercise
>
> A child has severe eczema that has not responded well to normal treatments. The parents insist on trying a complementary remedy recommended to them by a self-help group. How would you feel about this? What issues would you need to take account of? What are the implications for the therapeutic relationship?

Community nurses are required to demonstrate evidence-based practice (Woodward 2001) and the challenge of today's therapeutic relationship is to balance this with informed choice by the patient (Wilson 2002). There is a balance to be maintained between the rights of the child (dependant on their age and understanding) and rights of the parents in decision-making, against the risks of significant harm that might result from the treatment. The parents in the above scenario should be advised to ensure the advice regarding the complementary treatment comes from a registered practitioner. Community nurses need to assess their own knowledge base regarding complementary therapy and seek specialist advice if necessary. Within a therapeutic relationship the nurse will be aiming to facilitate an atmosphere where the parents feel able to be honest about the treatments the child is currently receiving, and should be able to direct patients and their families to sources of appropriate information.

A final feature of the current context of care that may have an effect on the therapeutic relationship is the fragmentation of care. In particular the division of health and social care (DOH 1990) means that patients within the community often have to deal with a vast array of professionals, which can inhibit the development of a therapeutic relationship (Hyde and Cotter 2001).

CONCLUSION

In this chapter features of a therapeutic relationship have been identified, leading to an exploration of some of the challenges community nurses face in establishing therapeutic relationships. In future community health care provision, challenges will be shaped by an increasingly multi-cultural, ageing and informed population. The growing provision of health care in the community only serves to reinforce the need to establish appropriate relationships with patients, their families and other carers. Current government policy emphasises partnership in care at all levels; the challenge for the community nurse is to develop this opportunity in everyday working practice.

FURTHER READING

Smith, P. (1992) *The Emotional Labour of Nursing*. Basingstoke: Macmillan.

REFERENCES

Aggleton, P. and Chalmers, H. (2000) *Nursing Models and Nursing Practice* (2nd edn). Basingstoke: Macmillan.

Atwell, C. (1996) Health in the workplace. In S. Twinn, B. Roberts, and S. Andrews (eds), *Community Health Care Nursing: Principles for Practice*. Oxford: Butterworth-Heinemann, 260–75.

Barnsteiner, J.H. and Gillis-Donovan, J. (1990) Being related and separated: a standard for therapeutic relationships. *Maternal Child Nursing Journal*, 15: 223–8.

Bond, J., Farrow, G. and Gregson, B.A. *et al.* (1999) Informal care-giving for frail older people at home and in long-term care institutions: who are the key supporters? *Health and Social Care in the Community*, 7(6): 434–4.

Brooker, C. and Repper, J. (eds) (1998) *Serious Mental Health Problems in the Community: Policy, Practice and Research*. London: Ballière Tindall.

Bryans, A. and McIntosh, J. (1996) Decision making in community nursing: an analysis of the stages of decision making as they relate to community nursing assessment practice. *Journal of Advanced Nursing*, 24: 24–30.

Chambers (1993) *The Chambers Dictionary*. Edinburgh: Chambers Harrap.

Collister, B. (1986) Psychiatric nursing and a developmental model. In B. Kershaw. and J. Salvage (eds), *Models for Nursing*. Chichester: John Wiley.

Copperman, J. and Morrison, P. (1995) *We Thought We Knew: Involving Patients in Nursing Practice*. London: King's Fund.

Crowe, M. (2000). The nurse–patient relationship: a consideration of its discursive context. *Journal of Advanced Nursing*, 31(4): 962–7.

Department of Health (1990) *The NHS and Community Care Act*. London: HMSO.

Department of Health (1995) *Carers Recognition and Services Act*. London: HMSO.

Department of Health (1999a) *National Service Framework for Mental Health*. London: The Stationery Office.

Department of Health (1999b) *Our Healthier Nation: Saving Lives*. London: The Stationery Office.

Department of Health (2000) *Carers and Disabled Children Act* London: HMSO.

Department of Health (2001a) *National Service Framework for Older People*. London: Department of Health.

Department of Health (2001b) *The Expert Patient: A New Approach to Chronic Disease Management for the 21st Century*. London: The Stationery Office.

Dukes Hess, J. (1996) The ethics of compliance: a dialectic. *Advances in Nursing Science*, 19(1): 18–27.

Feenan, D. (1997) Capable people: empowering the patient in the assessment of capacity. *Health Care Analysis*, 5(3): 227–36.

Goodman, C., Knight, D., Machen, I. and Hunt, B. (1998) Emphasizing terminal care as district nursing: a helpful strategy in a purchasing environment? *Journal of Advanced Nursing*, 28(3): 491–8.

Health and Safety Executive (2000) *Stress is a Workplace Issue – HSE begins Publicity Drive. Press Release E206:00*. London: HSE.

Henwood, M. (1998) *Ignored and invisible? Carers' Experience of the NHS*. London: Carers National Association.

Hyde, V. and Cotter, C. (2001) The development of community nursing in the light of the NHS Plan. In V. Hyde. (ed.), *Community Nursing and Health Care: Insights and Innovations*. London: Arnold.

Hylton Rushton, C., Armstrong, L. and McEnhill, M. (1996). Establishing therapeutic boundaries as patient advocates. *Pediatric Nursing*, 22(3): 185–9.

Jerome, A. and Ferraro-McDuffie, A. (1992) Nurse self awareness in therapeutic relationships, *Pediatric Nursing*, 18(2): 153–6.

Kalache, A. (1996): Ageing worldwide. In S. Ebrahim and A. Kalache (eds), *Epidemiology in Old Age*. London: BMJ Publishing Group.

Lorig, K., Stewart, A., Ritter, P. *et al.* (1996) *Outcome Measures for Health Education and Other Health Care Interventions*. Thousand Oaks, CA: Sage.

May, C. and Purkis, M.E. (1997) Editorial: exploring relationships between professionals, patients and others. *Health and Social Care in the Community*, 5(1): 1–2.

McMahon, R. and Pearson, A. (1998) *Nursing as Therapy* (2nd edn). Cheltenham: Stanley Thornes.

McParland, J. Scott, P. Arndt, M. *et al.* (2000) Autonomy and clinical practice, 1: identifying areas of concern. *British Journal of Nursing*, 9(8): 507–13.

Morse, J.M. (1991) Negotiating commitment and involvement in the nurse–patient relationship. *Journal of Advanced Nursing*, 16: 455–68.

Normandale, S. (2001) A study of mother's perceptions of the health visiting role. *Community Practitioner*, 74(4): 146–50.

Nursing and Midwifery Council (2002) *Code of Professional Conduct*. London: NMC.

Parkin, P. (2001) Covert community nursing: reciprocity in formal and informal relations. In Hyde, V. (ed.), *Community Nursing and Health Care: Insights and Innovations*. London: Arnold.

Paterson, B. (2001) Myth of empowerment in chronic illness. *Journal of Advanced Nursing*, 34(5): 574–81.

Peplau, H.E. (1952) *Interpersonal Relations in Nursing*. New York: Putnam.

Pickard, S., Shaw, S. and Glendinning, C. (2000) Health care professionals' support for older carers. *Ageing and Society*, 20: 725–44.

Procter, S., Wilcockson, J., Pearson, P. *et al.* (2001) Going home from hospital: the carer/patient dyad. *Journal of Advanced Nursing*, 35(2): 206–17.

Roberts, K. (2001) Across the health-social care divide: elderly people as active users of health care and social care. *Health and Social Care in the Community*, 9(2): 100–07.

Royal Pharmaceutical Society of Great Britain (1997) *Compliance to Concordance: Achieving Shared Goals in Medicine Taking*. London: RPSGB.

Seddon, D. and Robinson, C.A. (2001) Carers of older people with dementia: assessment and the *Carers Act. Health and Social Care in the Community*, 9(3): 151–8.

Timmons, S. (2001) Use of the Internet by patients: not a threat to nursing, but an opportunity? *Nurse Education Today*, 21(2): 104–9.

Totka, J. (1996) Exploring the boundaries of paediatric practice: nurse stories related to relationships. *Pediatric Nursing*, 22(3): 191–6.

Twigg, J. and Atkin, K. (1994) *Carers Perceived*. Buckingham: Open University.

United Kingdom Central Council (1999) *Practitioner–Client Relationships and the Prevention of Abuse*. London: UKCC.

Waterworth, S. and Luker, K.A. (1990) Reluctant collaborators: do patients want to be involved in decisions concerning care? *Journal of Advanced Nursing*, 15: 971–6.

Wellard, S. (1998) Constructions of chronic illness. *International Journal of Nursing Studies*, 35: 49–55.

Wilson, P.M. (2001a) *Being the Last Resort: A critical ethnography of district nurses and their patients with long-term needs*. Unpublished MSc thesis, University of Manchester, RCN Institute.

Wilson, P.M. (2001b) A policy analysis of the 'expert patient' in the United Kingdom: self-care as an expression of pastoral power? *Health and Social Care in the Community*, 9(3): 134–42.

Wilson, P.M. (2002) The expert patient: issues and implications for community nurses. *British Journal of Community Nursing*, 7(10): 514–19.

Woodward, V. (2001) Evidence-based practice, clinical governance and community nurses. In V. Hyde (ed.), *Community Nursing and Health Care: Insights and Innovations*. London: Arnold.

Working collaboratively

Ann Clarridge and Elaine Ryder

Learning outcomes

- An understanding of why collaborative working is so essential in terms of the government policy.
- An understanding of what is meant by collaboration.
- An appreciation of the issues relating to the interface of collaborative working.
- A recognition of the skills that are required in order to collaborate effectively.
- An acknowledgement of the interprofessional relations, including some of the barriers and constraints, that can affect collaborative working.

Collaborative working has become a significant feature of current and future practice. This chapter seeks to define collaboration and to explore a number of its different aspects. It includes the attitudes and skills required, the issues surrounding interprofessional relationships and some of the constraints and barriers that can arise. The aim is to assist those nurses who choose to work in primary care to understand more fully the complexities of care delivery within this setting. It will mention the range of professionals and agencies who work with patients to meet their needs.

INTRODUCTION

The ability to work collaboratively has been highlighted in the professional *Code of Conduct* (NMC 2002a) as an essential part of a nurse's role. There is an expectation that a nurse will work co-operatively with other professionals, respecting their skills, expertise and contributions. Additionally, a nurse must communicate effectively to share knowledge, skills and expertise in order to work efficiently with other team members, whilst maintaining high standards of care (NMC 2002a). Nurses who seek to enrich their practice need

to have a greater understanding of what it means to work collaboratively, not just with other professionals but primarily with patients and their carers (Fatchett 1996). This active involvement of patients in their care lies at the heart of current government policy (DOH 2001a, 2001b). Whilst the aim of collaborative working is that it should lead either to health gains or improved patient outcomes, it must be noted that there is, according to Ross and Mackenzie (1996), insufficient evidence to date to substantiate this view – an interesting finding given that policy and practice place such emphasis on collaborative working.

The following case study of a hypothetical family in receipt of primary care will be used to contextualise the issues being discussed.

Example

Elmer King, aged 35 years, is black British of Caribbean origin but grew up in London. He is unemployed, suffering from schizophrenia and carries sickle cell trait. His partner Ann, aged 32 years, is white British. She also carries sickle cell trait. She has a part-time night cleaning job for a large local firm.

Malcolm Roberts, aged 13 years, is the son of Ann's first partner. He is timid and small for his age. He 'gets picked on' by other children at school and has recently been complaining of stomach aches and not wanting to go to school.

Louise King, aged 8 years, has sickle cell disease and has had a lot of absence from school because of sickle cell crises.

Alice King, aged 11 months, is wheezy and suffers from severe infantile eczema. She was bottle-fed from birth and weaned very early. She has attended for developmental checks. Her hearing and vision are satisfactory but there is concern about delayed motor development.

Ann recently scalded her leg badly. She says she accidentally knocked over a full pot of freshly made tea. She has been self-treating the wound for a few days and has only just visited her general practitioner (GP) as the wound is now 'rather smelly' and her leg is very red.

The family live in an urban area of a large city. Their accommodation, which they rent, is a small terraced house with two bedrooms and a small garden at the rear.

In considering issues relating to Elmer, Ann and their family there is the potential for a number of different people to be involved in order to provide the appropriate services to meet the family's health and social needs.

IMPLICATIONS OF GOVERNMENT POLICY FOR COLLABORATION

Over the past 15 years, government health and social policy has constantly reinforced the need for primary health care and teamwork to meet the challenges of a changing population and of 'life-style related disease in the community' (Ross and Mackenzie 1996: p.78). In 1986 the Cumberlege Report (DHSS 1986) noted that numerous health and social care professionals were 'beating the same pathway' to patients. The results were confusion for the patients and their carers and duplication of services. It was considered that the service provision was fragmented and the potential for missing health needs was significant. Through a series of government policies (DOH 1987, 1989a, 1989b, 1990, 1996, 1997, 1999a, 1999b), teamwork, collaboration and a partnership approach to care have become central to the provision of care in the community. There is recognition of a need to move away from the traditional boundaries of health and social care towards the development of multi-professional teams working throughout hospital and primary care settings.

The NHS and Community Care Act 1990 brought together the social services and health services to provide 'seamless care' to people in their own homes or in homely settings. The Act provided a 'planning framework' to enable different agencies to work together, to consult and collaborate at every level (Audit Commission 1992). This 'bringing together' was further strengthened in the subsequent government report, *Primary Care-Led NHS* (DOH 1996). It was envisaged that multi-disciplinary, multi-professional, inter-agency teams of people would be working together. In a time of diminishing resources and increasing demand they would provide an effective, high-quality care that would be needs led and not merely a blanket provision.

It was the change of government in 1997 that brought about recent changes of policy in the National Health Service, but the need for partnership and collaborative working has remained a significant feature – in fact has been emphasised more strongly. One of six key underpinning principles outlined in *The New NHS: Modern, Dependable* (DOH 1997) was to involve the National Health Service in partnership with other agencies in the provision of social and health care, with the needs of the patient at the centre of the care process. The increasing emphasis on the role of primary health care teams has come about as a result of ever-increasing hospital costs alongside government recognition of their importance as gate-keepers to health care (Fatchett 1996). The more recent *NHS Plan* (DOH 2000) has contributed to this shift in emphasis to a needs-led service – one that encompasses collaboration, joint working and partnership. Fatchett (1996) has attributed the increase in popularity to collaboration to a number of causes.

- A growth in the complexity of health and welfare services.
- Expansion of knowledge and subsequent increase in specialisation.
- A perceived need for the rationalisation of resources.
- A need to reduce the duplication of care.
- The provision of a more effective, integrated and supportive service for both users and professionals.

The greater complexity of technology and treatment has placed tremendous pressure upon practitioners to have the necessary knowledge and competencies to meet the needs of patients with complex care needs. There have been a number of recent public inquiries into incidents involving people who have been diagnosed as mentally ill. Government response has been to seek to improve the co-ordination of care for such individuals, with an increased emphasis on the role of the primary health care teams (Secker *et al.* 2000).

without reference to the patients and their carers. Interestingly enough, the issue about being professionally driven could be inferred from policy documentation (DOH 1992). Here collaboration is seen as a 'partnership of individuals and organisations formed to enable people to increase their influence over the factors that affect their health and well being', a view more recently expressed in *The NHS Plan* (DOH 2000) and *Liberating the Talents* (DOH 2002).

The issue of collaboration having the potential to be professionally driven is of particular importance when considering a partnership approach between practitioners, patients and their carers. Henneman *et al.* (1995) suggest that when individuals are involved in collaboration their relationship is non-hierarchical. Power is shared on the basis of knowledge and expertise rather than role or title. In other words, collaborative working needs to involve a redistribution of power within the health care team (Soothill *et al.*1995).

> ## Exercise
>
> Which agencies might be involved in supporting Elmer, Ann and their family?

> ## Exercise
>
> Collaborative working can be seen as a multi-faceted concept. Identify the skills and knowledge needed by the practitioners for effective collaborative working.

DEFINING COLLABORATION

As highlighted in the previous section, the reasons given for collaborative working would seem to be extensive and significant, but what does it actually mean? The word 'collaborate' is derived from the Latin *collaborare* which means 'to labour together'. This notion of working together has been highlighted by Ovretveit (1997) in the sense of collaboration between organisations or individuals working together or acting jointly. In addition, the notion of exchange is evident in Armitage's definition (1983), defining collaboration as being the exchange of information between individuals involved in the delivery of care, which has the potential for action or joint working in the interests of a common purpose.

This definition would seem to be quite straightforward, but it could also be seen to be referring exclusively to professionals delivering care

THE INTERFACE OF COLLABORATIVE CARE

In considering the needs of Elmer, Ann and their family there will be a need to relate to and work with each member of the family as well as networking with a range of diverse groups, including social services, and voluntary agencies. The interface may be at different levels, according to the actual requirements of care. Armitage (1983) identified a taxonomy of levels of collaboration that moves from a situation where people communicate without meeting to a situation where people work together. For example, issues of child protection and bullying that could be associated with Alice and Malcolm might be dealt with by the health visitor and the school nurse, who might also involve such other agencies as social workers, the police and the judiciary. The GP and the practice nurse may be involved with the care of Ann's wound and for Elmer's maintenance medication. In this way referrals from one agency to another regarding the family might occur without any need for a meeting. However, if the care is to be effective it might be that each of the agencies involved would need to come together and meet with the family to resolve difficulties, duplication and problems. Similarly, two agencies might be more involved than others and take the lead in the care whilst informing the remaining agencies of progress.

A framework for classifying collaboration by Gray (1989, cited in Huxham 1996) suggests that there are two dimensions: factors that motivate people to collaborate and the goal or anticipated outcome of the collaboration. Gray further suggested that there are four types of collaboration: appreciative planning, dialogues, collective strategies and negotiated settlements. Although Gray is concerned specifically with business organisations, her classification of the four types of collaboration could also be applied to health care situations.

The different types of collaboration as identified by Gray can be seen at a micro level, as in the King family. The exchange of information is one of the key features in the King family's situation (*appreciative planning*). Each of the different practitioners involved with Elmer, Ann and the family care need to communicate (*dialogues)* their knowledge of the situation in order to arrive at a shared vision. They need to provide an arena for exploring solutions to the problems identified by the patients and their carers, resolve difficulties (*negotiated settlements*) and reach agreement about a plan of care (*collective strategies*). Thus the collaborative process will pass through three phases: problem solving, direction setting and implementation (Gray 1989, cited in Huxham 1996).

At a broader macro level, working in partnership and collaborative care means ensuring that the structure of the organisation is sufficiently flexible to support patients and enable them to function. The implementation of health improvement programmes (HIPs) is seen as providing the 'strategic glue' that binds the different services together in new working partnerships between users and health service providers, including statutory and non-statutory (Gillam and Irvine 2000). In addressing the needs of local populations through HIPs there is an emphasis upon primary care staff to work across practice and professional boundaries with colleagues in Social Services, Education and Housing. In this way, people with the relevant knowledge and skill, including the patients and their carers, will be able to carry out the appropriate care.

> ### Exercise
>
> If the King family were on your caseload, what processes would you need to establish to meet their needs?

SKILLS NEEDED TO COLLABORATE EFFECTIVELY

Previous sections of this chapter have discussed why it is important to work collaboratively, what it means to collaborate and with whom we need to collaborate. This section is about how we collaborate – in particular the skills needed to collaborate effectively. Using the case study of Elmer, Ann and their family, scenarios will be drawn out to demonstrate the range of skills that are fundamental to effective collaboration.

Hornby and Atkins (2000) are clear in establishing that the sole purpose of collaboration is to provide optimum help. In their discussion on collaborative processes and problems, they identified a range of attitudes and skills necessary for good practice. It is these that will be identified and integrated in an examination of this complex family situation.

Thompson (1996) states that working with others involves engaging with other people person-to-person. However, before we can do this we have to have a good understanding of ourselves in terms of 'how we are perceived by other people, our characteristic responses and reaction and our own needs' (p. 234).

Collaborative attitudes

Hornby and Atkins (2000) suggest that collaborative attitudes may be clustered under the concepts: *reciprocity, flexibility* and *integrity*.

- *Reciprocity* is based on respect and concern for individuals and the development of mutual understanding and mutual trust.
- *Flexibility* is the readiness to explore new ideas and methods of practice and an open attitude to change. It is about working in partnership with clients and colleagues and not about positions of power.
- *Professional integrity* places the client's needs first and not those of the individual practitioner. Integrity, according to Hornby and Atkins, demands that practitioners examine their own defensive practices and separatist tendencies.

Exercise

Consider what reciprocity, flexibility and professional integrity would mean in relation to the following scenario.

Elmer usually attends the health centre for his regular depot injections from the practice nurse. He has not attended for the second injection and the nurse is very concerned about Elmer. She has tried to contact him by telephone but the number is unobtainable – in fact it has been cut off due to non-payment of bills.

This scenario highlights the importance of collaborative attitudes. In considering the issues of reciprocity, flexibility and professional integrity, you may have covered the following issues.

Reciprocity. The practice nurse has shown genuine concern and empathy for Elmer. She has begun to build up a relationship with him during his routine appointments and her knowledge of his condition has led her to feel genuine concern. In the busy schedule demanded by the appointment system at the surgery, it would be easy to label Elmer as a 'DNA' (did not attend) and be somewhat dismissive of any follow-up. Mutual trust is beginning to develop between the practice nurse and Elmer and the fact that she has been unable to contact him on the phone, has led her to feel that 'something is wrong'.

Flexibility. The practice nurse has shown by her actions that she sees Elmer as an equal partner in his care. Her approach is one of working towards concordance (see DOH 2001a) as opposed to compliance. She would be keen to consider other methods of practice, depending on Elmer's needs.

Professional integrity. The practice nurse has demonstrated the importance she places on meeting Elmer's needs – it would have been easy for her to become irritated by Elmer's 'DNA'. In terms of her role within the practice and the other patients she has been more prepared to consider what is wrong with Elmer than her own position at that time. However, she should also realise that she is not alone in being able to provide support for Elmer. She is a member of a wider primary health care team, some of whom might be better placed to follow up Elmer's situation. In this way she would be demonstrating her awareness of her own role and its boundaries whilst respecting the roles of the others in the team.

Exercise

Who do you think the practice nurse could collaborate with regarding Elmer's situation?

Elmer's community mental health nurse would probably be the first colleague to contact regarding his schizophrenia and depot medication. She might also want to discuss the situation with her health visitor colleague, who would know the family because of visiting Ann and baby Alice. Both these colleagues would be able to discuss Elmer's financial situation with him and seek further support from the social worker, should he wish it. She could also contact the school nurse responsible for the schools that Louise and Malcolm attend just to ensure that the children have the opportunity to share any concerns if they wish and to monitor their situation.

In summary, this scenario demonstrates how important it is to have a positive attitude to collaboration not only with patients but also with colleagues.

Collaborative skills

In addition to collaborative attitudes, Hornby and Atkins (2000) highlight the importance of collaborative skills and see these as *relational*, *organising* and *assessment skills* – all essential elements for effective collaborative working.

Relational skills include *open listening, empathy, communicating* and *a helping manner*, in other words putting people at their ease.

Open listening means hearing without stereotyping, and using direction purely for the purpose of hearing more rather than less. It requires the ability to tolerate distress and anxiety without resorting to coping methods that restrict the client's communications. It means being alert to the feelings that may be involved when individuals seek and receive help and being aware of the effect on people of finding themselves as a service user. It is about facilitating the expression of relevant emotions and being able to empathise whilst at the same time retaining the necessary objectivity when meeting patients' needs.

Empathy, according to Thompson (1996), is the ability to appreciate the feelings and circumstances of others even though we do not necessarily share them. It is about being sensitive to differences and avoiding making stereotypical assumptions. In order to avoid discrimination and disadvantage, it is essential that patients' differing requirements are met.

Clements and Spinks (1994) stress the importance of treating others, whether as individuals or in groups, fairly, sensitively and with courtesy, regardless of who they may be. Further, they identify the following skills, knowledge and attitudes, which are applicable to almost any situation:

- empathy
- keeping within the law
- thinking about the consequences
- not believing myths
- a desire to be fair
- openness to different ideas
- reflective thinking
- sensitivity
- using appropriate language
- knowing about the issues
- treating people as individuals
- not seeing alternative cultures as a threat.

Open communicating means conveying what seems to be relevant, including feelings as well as facts and opinions, without becoming defensive. Where trust is lacking, defensive processes and protective devices are likely to come into operation. Open communicating also relates to the need for professional confidentiality (NMC 2002b). For further information about confidentiality see Cornock (2001).

A helping manner, according to Hornby and Atkins (2000), is the ability to manifest personal concern and professional confidence without superiority, thus enabling patients, carers and practitioners to function at their best in a working relationship. The role of carers should not be taken for granted nor undervalued: the practitioner must be as concerned for their wellbeing as for that of the patient. This feeling of being valued may not automatically result in an increased participation but it can at least bring emotional benefit to both carer and patient. Facilitating patients' and carers' expressions of their feelings is a skill which can often increase understanding of a situation, resolve blocks to progress and relieve tension and distress.

Exercise

In terms of relational skills, for example open listening, communication and a helping manner, what do you feel are some of the issues in the following scenario?

The district nurse has received a referral from the GP regarding visiting Mrs King, who has recently scalded her leg. She has been self-treating the wound for several days and it has now become infected. The district nurse has not had any previous contact with Mrs King.

Mrs King has a night-time cleaning job for a large local supermarket and with her family commitments is not able to attend the health centre. The district nurse knocks hard on the door and eventually Mrs King appears in her nightie, looking cross. She was asleep and Elmer, who should have been looking after baby Alice, has gone out.

You may have considered some of the following points. At the initial referral it would have been helpful if the GP had indicated that Mrs King worked 'nights'. Even though she could not confirm her visit by telephone the district nurse should have been able to make a visit at a time more convenient for Mrs King which intruded less on her need to sleep during the day. It might have averted the initial 'angry' meeting. However, once in this somewhat confrontational position, the district nurse needs to be able to acknowledge the situation as a whole and her role in it. She needs to be receptive to Mrs King's irritation and demonstrate her open listening skills. It would be easy to become defensive and use closed questions as a means of restricting Mrs King's communication. Skills in open communication are essential in order to build a trusting relationship between practitioner and patient. A helping manner is demonstrated by concern for the individual patient within the wider family context. This example shows how important it is for the practitioner to view a situation from a holistic perspective rather than from a limited task viewpoint. In an uncomfortable atmosphere the practitioner could well have undertaken a specific task and then left, limiting her concern solely to Mrs King's leg.

Organising skills identified by Hornby and Atkins (2000) are those required to implement the principles of essential collaboration. These include establishing networks, setting up meetings, devising appropriate patient/carer referral systems, and managing changes within the work context. Professional boundaries need to be clearly defined and agreed. Henneman *et al.* (1995) maintain that collaboration requires individuals to have both a clear understanding of their own role and an understanding and respect for the roles of others.

When individual team members are clear about their own roles and boundaries and those of others in the team, the most appropriate person can then support Elmer and his family – otherwise gaps in their support could appear. The complex situation presented by Elmer's family requires an effective application of skills. The family, the GP, practice nurse, receptionist, community mental health nurse, district nurse and school nurse have already been indicated as each having a role to play. Clearly, networking with others in such a situation is crucial. The primary health care team meeting

could prove to be a valuable forum where issues would be shared, future support for the family clarified, and the key worker identified. A lack of organisational skills could prevent a full and accurate picture of the family's needs being completed.

Assessment skills represent the final element of collaborative skills as identified by Hornby and Atkins (2000). Assessment, according to Thompson (1996), is a complex and multi-faceted process. A high level of interpersonal skills is required when undertaking a holistic assessment, and in complex situations assessment skills involving a range of perspectives may be appropriate. When different agencies have overlapping boundaries sometimes the patient can experience difficulty in finding that which is most suited to meeting his/her needs. At the same time it is not always possible for one practitioner to have sufficient in-depth knowledge of the various contributions of other agencies. Practitioners need to know enough about a range of services to be able to select the most appropriate one for any given situation and also when to refer the patient. Thus, the demands on the practitioner include not only a wide range of knowledge and a high level of assessment skills but also a freedom from defensive or separatist attitudes (Hornby and Atkins 2000). Whilst there is a desire to move towards a single assessment process, currently different professionals have their own methods for documenting assessment (NMC 2002b). It is the pooling of this information that is so important to ensure that all the pieces of information fit together.

INTERPROFESSIONAL RELATIONS

The final section of this chapter focuses on interprofessional relationships, thus drawing together some of the wider issues already alluded to.

Exercise

Within your area of practice, identify a complex family situation and identify potential barriers and constraints to collaborative working.

Mackay *et al.* (1995) have asserted that working interprofessionally involves crossing traditional professional boundaries, being prepared to be flexible in considering a range of views and having a willingness to listen to what colleagues from other disciplines are saying. Each group brings different skills and solutions to the health care problem with which they are presented. In some decisions the contribution of one professional group needs to take precedence over others, which underlines the need for flexibility in decision making. Interprofessional working, as mentioned earlier, raises the question of redistribution of power within teams. So many fundamental changes are taking place within primary care that perhaps now is an opportune moment to challenge established and entrenched attitudes.

Collaboration between professionals and between service agencies is currently regarded as the cornerstone of the development of community care in the UK. However, only recently have mechanisms of collaboration been subject to evaluation as a means of demonstrating effectiveness. Molyneux (2001) attempted to do just this in her study of interprofessional team-working by identifying and evaluating the positive characteristics of team working. Three main themes emerged:

- *Motivation and flexibility of staff.* Personal qualities of staff such as flexibility, adaptability and lack of professional jealousy enabled team members to work across professional boundaries.
- *Communication within the team.* Findings identified regular and frequent team meetings and agreement on the communication strategies, for example shared records, within the team as central to effective team working.
- *Opportunities for creative development of working frameworks.* Encouragement and opportunities need to be provided for staff working together to enable them to develop creative methods of working which meets their patients' needs.

It is in the sharing of knowledge and skills in a collaborative way that the common goal of holistic care is more likely to be achieved with ultimate benefits to the patient and family. (Shields *et al.* 1995). Essential to the success of collaborative working is a defined mechanism for making

decisions. Problems can occur where a team does not have a clear and agreed process. Ovretveit (1993) points out that conflict can arise unless differences are aired and worked through in a creative and fair way. Unstructured decision making procedures waste time, cause conflict and resentment and can lead to team break down.

In summary, collaborative working is an ideal that essentially seeks to ensure that the best interests of the patient are protected. It is a never-ending process in which the patient, relatives and carers must increasingly be supported to play a central role in making their own contribution to decisions affecting their lives. Collaborative working is, therefore, one step on the way to fully informed decision making in meeting the needs of patients and their carers and delivering effective and efficient community health care.

REFERENCES

Armitage, N.H. (1983) Joint working in primary health care. *Nursing Times*, 79:75–8.

Audit Commission (1992) *Homeward bound: A New Course for Community Health.* London: HMSO.

Clements, P. and Spinks, T. (1994) *The Equal Opportunities Guide.* London: Kogan Page.

Cornock, M.A. (2001) Ethical and legal considerations of community nursing. In V. Hyde (ed.), *Community Nursing and Health Care.* London: Arnold.

Department of Health (1987) *Promoting Better Health.* London: HMSO.

Department of Health (1989a) *Working for Patients.* London: HMSO.

Department of Health (1989b) *Caring for People.* London: HMSO.

Department of Health (1990) *The NHS and Community Care Act.* London: HMSO.

Department of Health (1992) *The Health of the Nation.* London: HMSO.

Department of Health (1996) *A Primary Care-Led NHS.* London: HMSO.

Department of Health (1997) *The New NHS: Modern, Dependable.* London: The Stationery Office.

Department of Health (1999a) *Saving Lives.* London: The Stationery Office.

Department of Health (1999b) *Making a Difference.* London: The Stationery Office.

Department of Health (2000) *The NHS Plan.* London: The Stationery Office.

Department of Health (2001a) *Shifting the Balance of Power.* London: The Stationery Office.

Department of Health (2001b) *The Expert Patient.* London: The Stationery Office.

Department of Health (2002) *Liberating the Talents.* London: The Stationery Office.

Department of Health and Social Security (1986) *Neighbourhood Nursing: A Focus for Care* (Cumberlege report). London: HMSO.

Fatchett, A. (1996) A chance for community nurses to shape the health agenda. *Nursing Times*, 92: 40–2.

Gerrish, K. (1999) Teamwork in primary care: an evaluation of the contribution of integrated nursing teams. *Health and Social Care in the Community*, 7(5): 367–75.

Gillam, S. and Irvine, S. (2000) Editorial: Collaboration in the new NHS. *Journal of Interprofessional Care*, 14(1): 5–7.

Gray, B. (1989) *Collaborating: Finding Common Ground for Multiparty Problems.* San Francisco, CA: Jossey-Bass.

Henneman, E.A., Lee, J.L. and Cohen, J.I. (1995) Collaboration: a concept analysis. *Journal of Advanced Nursing*, 21:103–9.

Huxham, C. (1996) *Creating Collaborative Advantage* (1st edn). London: Sage.

Hornby, S. and Atkins, J. (2000) *Collaborative Care.* Oxford: Blackwell Science.

Mackay, L., Soothill, K. and Webb, C. (1995) Troubled times: the context for interprofessional collaboration. In Soothill, K.L., Mackay, L. and Webb, C. (eds) *Interprofessional Relations in Health Care.* London: Arnold.

Molyneux J. (2001) Interprofessional teamworking: what makes teams work well? *Journal of Interprofessional Care*, 15(1): 29–35.

Nursing Midwifery Council (2002a) *Code of Conduct.* London: NMC.

Nursing Midwifery Council (2002b) *Guidelines for Records and Record Keeping.* London: NMC.

Ovretveit, J. (1993) *Co-ordinating Community Care.* Buckingham: Open University Press.

Ovretveit, J. (1997) *Interprofessional Working for Health and Social Care.* London: Macmillan.

Ross, F. and Mackenzie, A. (1996) *Nursing in Primary Health Care Policy into Practice.* London: Routledge.

Secker, J., Pidd, F., Parham, A. and Peck, E. (2000) Mental health in the community: roles, responsibilities and organisation of primary care and specialist services. *Journal of Interprofessional Care*, 14(1): 49–58.

Shields, G., Hoelzle, L. and Schondel, C. (eds) (1995) Social work and nursing collaboration: a case study in assessing and meeting patient and family needs. *Journal of Interprofessional Care*, 9(1):21–9.

Soothill, K., Mackay, L. and Webb, C. (eds) (1995) *Interprofessional Relations in Health Care.* London: Arnold.

Thompson, N. (1996) *People Skills.* London; Macmillan.

7

Conceptual approaches to care

Milly Smith

Learning outcomes

- Discuss the underlying principles from which nursing care is developed.
- Explore the meaning of conceptual approaches to care.
- Explore conceptual approaches that are in common use in community nursing.
- Discuss and critically apply the concept of evidence-based practice to aspects of community nursing.
- Review the concept of reflection as a means of learning and establish as a concepts of sound practice.

INTRODUCTION

The term 'nursing model' was probably introduced to you in your basic education, and used for assignment work. Nursing models are supposed to be used in practice but in reality they are generally not used well, and appear to serve more as checklists for care plans rather than to inform the direction of nursing care. You may now be questioning the value of models of nursing, if they are simply used as a theoretical exercise in nurse education and a checklist in routine practice, but nursing models can, properly used, facilitate thinking about care and the philosophy that underpins it.

Most nurses have used one or more nursing models. You are likely to be familiar with the Activities of Living model (Roper, Logan and Tierney 1980, 2000) and the Self Care model (Orem 1971, 1991). There are many models that can inform nursing and health practice. Models are not simple; they have been very rigorously contemplated by experts and each one serves as a representation of nursing. An interesting point about nursing models is the way in which they vary quite considerably, so that the purpose and intention of one, and the way in which it informs

nursing, is quite different from these aspects in another model, and each is helpful to different branches of nursing. This will be discussed as the chapter develops.

Exercise

Think of a particular patient you have seen for the first time recently and use this person for the all the exercises in this chapter.

Imagine for a moment that models had never been developed. How would nurses approach patient care, what would inform actions and decisions in everyday practice?

You may or may not have been the first person to assess your patient's health state. If you were your decisions and actions about the care of the patient will be fundamental to all care following the initial assessment. Spend a few minutes considering what influenced the decisions that you made. It would be helpful to write down your ideas.

PHILOSOPHIES OF CARE

It is unlikely that anyone has a blank sheet, mentally, when approaching patient care, and this indicates that professionals take a considered approach in this matter. There are several labels for these general approaches. One approach to nursing is known as *task-orientated* – referring to the clinical task being carried out in isolation from any other aspects that influence the patient's condition. Thus the nurse dresses the wound and does not consider other factors that could influence the healing of the wound or the patient's comfort. Most nurses have heard the term *biomedical model*, which refers to treating the medical condition of the patient in isolation from the patient as a person. For instance, the patient's heart condition would be treated but their excess weight and sedentary lifestyle, and the anxiety they might have about their health, would be ignored. Pearson *et al.* (1996) consider that many nurses still use the biomedical model as the basis for their practice.

A term that is often used in relation to a general philosophy of care is *holistic*. The holistic approach takes into account a range of physiological and personal considerations for each individual and also places them in the context of contemporary society and of current health care provision. Holism is concerned with balance, i.e. with balancing the physical, psychosocial, and economic relationships of the person, with the environment in which they live (Aggleton and Chalmers 2000). Some branches of nursing, for example the nursing of those with learning disabilities, are more likely to take a holistic approach, as clients are not perceived in terms of a medical condition.

The underlying philosophy of our approach to nursing very much reflects our individuality. 'Philosophy' refers to the beliefs and values that shape the way each of us thinks and acts. You will certainly have heard the word used in the context of philosophy to life. Some common sayings exemplify such philosophies: Live now pay later; A short life but a good one; You reap what you sow. These sayings demonstrate our use of the term philosophy in this context: how our beliefs and values shape thinking and influence actions. It is to be expected that life experiences, education, professional socialisation and professional experience will shape a nurse's philosophy of care. Thus our underlying philosophy of care says something about us as individuals with unique personal experience.

Exercise

Put your personal philosophy of nursing into words and take a few minutes to consider some of the experiences that have influenced this philosophy.

Work out which general approach your philosophy reflects: does it reflect a biomedical or a holistic model?

CONCEPTUAL MODELS

Nurse theorists have examined the concept of nursing and have illustrated their ideas through nursing models. The full term is 'conceptual model', differentiating this kind of model from the sort that are exact miniatures of real objects – model cars, boats, buildings, for example. Each of these can be perfectly recreated as a working model. Is it possible to build such a model of nursing? The answer is, of course, No; and the reason for this is that nursing is a concept. A concept is a collection of images and ideas that help to classify things and it is not possible to build anything material from images and ideas. The notion of a concept can be explained through something that is familiar, for example the concept of spring. There are certain aspects that embody spring: lambs, daffodils, buds on trees, sunshine and warmer days. Put all these together and a set of images that creates a picture of the season of spring comes to mind. Nursing is a concept that is built around a set of images.

Exercise

Stop for a minute and consider what the concept of nursing suggests to you.

Your concept may involve images about caring, knowledge about health and illness, prevention of ill health, rehabilitation and enabling people to help themselves, partnerships with patients and other health workers, the list goes on. When nursing is viewed in this way it is easy to determine why models of nursing are conceptual. It would be impossible to build such a set of images into a visible working model.

It is possible to see that models may differ quite considerably because nurses think differently and hold divergent views about the concept. The difference in views will also reflect the varied concepts that are embodied in the different specialities of nursing. Take, for example, the conceptual difference between mental health and acute nursing. The concepts that make up the two roles will vary because the nature of nursing is different in each role; mental health nursing treating psychological disorders and imbalances while acute nursing is concerned with physical illness or disability. As conceptual models are developed for the nursing role it is logical that they will differ in accordance with the differences between branches of nursing.

Fawcett (1984) identified some common ground by analysing four key concepts that are embodied in all nursing models. These are: (1) the person or individual; (2) the environment in which nursing takes place; (3) health; and (4) nursing itself. Whatever other concepts make up a particular model, these four are found in all. Nurse theorists have attempted to build conceptual models that illustrate 'systematically constructed, scientifically based, and logically related sets of concepts which identify the essential components of nursing practice' (Riehl and Roy 1980: p. 6).

Building nursing models

Models must be put down in writing/text to enable them to be shared and used by other nurses. It is in this state that you have probably encountered nursing models. You might imagine how difficult it is to represent a complex set of concepts in writing. All models require to be portrayed through the written word and with the use of diagrams.

Before any model can be effectively used it must be interpreted and understood. It may take time to work through some of the terminology, but this is necessary if the is model to be used as intended. You

can see that Orem's model (1980) is based on the ability of people to care for themselves. The model represents a balance between what people need to be able to do, which Orem refers to as 'universal self care needs' and a person's ability to perform their care, which Orem refers to as 'self care'. The model also lists areas where, for various reasons, an individual may require nursing intervention and suggests, under methods of helping, the form that such intervention might take.

The model proposed by Orem has several components that relate to self care, starting with the premise that individuals wish to be independent and listing areas where people normally meet their own self care needs. There are health-related reasons that interfere with people's ability to be independent and to care for themselves. The model looks at general reasons why a person may need help and makes suggestions about ways in which a nurse may support a patient in their striving for self care. The overall philosophy is to support self care and independence, and this sets the tone of this particular model and the direction that nursing care will take.

Representing this conceptual model is not easy and Orem supports the concepts embodied in the model with detailed explanatory text. To use any model well, the whole model should be applied, with all concepts captured, in its application to patient care. Nurses tend to take what they consider to be the useful ideas from models and apply them in isolation. A prime example of this is the use of the Activities of Living model (Roper, Logan and Tierney, 1980, 2000), where the list of daily living activities is used as a checklist against which care plans are developed. This action ignores the essence of the model.

Exercise

It would help you at this point to refer to a text that deals explicitly with nursing models and explore Orem's model to understand general philosophical approach and the particular features of the model.

You should now have an understanding of the nature and purpose of a nursing model. One or more models should be used by a care team to guide the process of care, and the model(s) must be supported by all members. The team leader has responsibility to ensure that all team members are sufficiently knowledgeable to be able to use the chosen model(s) competently to follow through the planned programme of care. Effective caring using a nursing model is a team effort.

Exercise

Consider if and how Orem's Self Care model could be used for the patient you have in mind.

Models with differing philosophies

You may not feel that a Self Care model is suitable for the patient that you have in mind or for your branch of nursing. There are other options to explore, some similar to the ideas expressed in Orem's model, others very different. A similar model was developed by Roper, Logan and Tierney (1980, 2000), informed by earlier work from Henderson, who offered a definition of nursing based on 14 activities of daily living (Henderson 1966). The Activities of Living model is well known and much used in the British Isles. It approaches nursing care by considering the activities of living that are common to all people, and how these can be influenced by a range of factors, the origins of which might be physical, psychological, social, cultural, environmental, political or economic. Other aspects that come into the model are the age of the person and the degree to which they are able to lead an independent life. The model focuses strongly on the many factors that influence activities of daily living and requires nurses to take these into consideration in making judgements about nursing care.

Self care and activities of living tend to be concerned with planning nursing care in order to meet physical health deficits, which is why these two models are widely used to nurse patients with acute and chronic illnesses. They are equally suitable for wider use. Aggleton and Chalmers (2000) illustrate this point by applying the Activities of Living model to bereavement.

Other models take a very different philosophical approach. Roy (1976) proposed a model based on adaptation. It works from the premise that each person is constantly adapting to an ever-changing environment. Roy suggests that an altered state of health requires a person to adapt to cope with changed circumstances. She sees the role of the nurse as one of facilitating adaptation in the patient by adopting a systematic series of actions, directed towards the goals of adaptation. The role of the nurse in this model is to facilitate the patient to adapt to their altered health circumstances and through adaptation learn to cope with the change. This explanation is much over-simplified but it indicates yet another conceptual approach.

Neuman's Systems model (Neuman 1989) takes a very different conceptual approach, based on wellness. It is concerned with the patient's response to stressors in the environment. Each person develops a range of responses to cope with normal circumstances, with some people appearing to cope better than others with everyday life. There are, however, situations that occur in the lives of all people that deviate from normal and produce stressors that are very difficult to cope with. Neuman defines stressors as inert forces that have the ability to impact on the patient's steady state (Neuman 1989: pp. 12, 24). Some situations may be positive and enabling whilst others may be detrimental. This model views the nurse's role as intervening to enable the patient to maintain an optimal state of wellness. There may be opportunities in primary care practice to capitalise on facilitation and enable the patient to manage stressors that face them in order to attain an optimum state of health. Such a model may be well suited for use in school nursing, health visiting and occupational therapy.

In Peplau's Interpersonal Relations model (Peplau 1988) the key components are the interpersonal process, nurse, patient and anxiety. Peplau considers that people are motivated towards self-maintenance, reproduction and growth by biological, psychological and social qualities. The model views the interpersonal relationship between nurse and patient as the focal point of interface that will produce benefits for the patient's health. There are elements of adaptation and coping in this model with the main thrust of nursing intervention coming through the nurse–patient relationship as a therapeutic interpersonal process. A model such as this, based on interpersonal relationships, may be well suited to mental health and learning disability nursing.

The conceptual models that have been mentioned in this chapter serve to illustrate the wide and varying approaches that contribute to the development of models of nursing. The differing approaches afford choice in decisions that are taken about delivery of care, and consideration should be given by the care team to the most suitable choice of model for the patient. The models are complex and to use any one effectively it will be necessary to refer to texts where the model under consideration is fully examined. It will also be necessary to make sure that others involved in the care know and understand the model in all its aspects.

THE NURSING PROCESS: A MEANS OF IMPLEMENTING NURSING MODELS

The vehicle for implementing a nursing model is the nursing process, a functional approach to the organisation of nursing care. Yura and Walsh (1967) identified a number of stages in nursing care with which all nurses have some familiarity: assess, plan, implement, evaluate. The four stages of the process are used in conjunction with a nursing model and its philosophy. Using Orem's model as an example, the four stages of the nursing process could be applied as follows.

The *assessment stage* of the nursing process would take into consideration:

- the philosophy that people are normally self caring
- the ability of people to care for themselves, using universal self-care needs to guide the assessment
- recognition of the reasons an individual may require nursing intervention
- recognition of the way in which lifestyle and the patient's environment influence the situation.

The *care plan* would detail:

- the actions that need to be taken to meet identified needs in relation to the patient's normal lifestyle and wishes

- interventions that could be used to achieve self care, whether they are the responsibility of the nurse, the patient or others
- the type of intervention needed: for example, teaching how to carry out care, or giving care, and providing aids to living that enable the patient to regain independence
- ways in which the planned actions would be evaluated.

The *planned care* would then be given (implemented), bearing in mind that:

- planned care is given according to good practice;
- current knowledge that is evidence-based underpins the care
- lifestyle and the environment are accommodated in the provision of care
- care given is evaluated against changes in the patient's physical, psychological and socio-economic condition.

Evaluation of care takes place to determine its effectiveness. This is:

- carried out as an ongoing practice at each visit
- includes, at regular predetermined intervals, an objective review of the care with reference to changes in condition, treatment effectiveness, introduction of new treatments
- leads to an adjustment of the care plan, if necessary, updating it in accordance with the evidence of the review.

Thus the nursing process, systematically applying a model, connects theory to what is done on a practical level; and the nursing process and model(s) of care offer a care team a more supportive structure than can be provided by a task-oriented approach to nursing. They enable systematic, logical organisation of care to be developed around a philosophical focus.

Though we are here referring to 'nursing process', in fact the four-stage process outlined above can be applied to any situation that requires organising. It is a tool that can be just as useful for organising a charity walk or planning a teaching session.

Through the use of models of nursing and the nursing process there is good support on which to base nursing and health care practice, in a well planned manner. All nurses must be thoroughly conversant with models and process, but although these provide a philosophy of care and give structure to care, what else is needed to provide sound practice? Evidence from patient surveys suggests that patients would want competent and caring practitioners (Carey and Posovac 1982) and the next part of this chapter is concerned with competent practice.

EVIDENCE–BASED PRACTICE (EBP)

Exercise

Think again about your patient. How do you know that what you are doing is correct? Where do you acquire the evidence on which you base your nursing practice?

You are taught in formal and informal situations. You read professional journals, books, literature from medical suppliers and drug companies. You observe those who you work with, some of whom you admire as role models. As you progress through your career you gain from experience. Many things that you have done have worked well and the patient has had positive outcomes from your care. These positive outcomes are sources of learning: you learned from something that went well. Learning can also take place following a poor experience. If something did not work well or went wrong a great deal can be gained from reflecting on the event, identifying what went wrong and considering measures that could be taken to improve the situation.

Objectivity in nursing practice

Learning takes place in a variety of ways and everyday work provides a mixture of objective and subjective learning experiences. Information that is evidence-based has been based on research studies, and this is objective knowledge, gained from systematically established evidence. Subjective knowledge is gathered from observations made in practice, from conversations with colleagues and sometimes from teaching sessions. The problem with knowledge gained in this way is that it may not

be reliable, and could even be unsound and dangerous. It is important that care is planned on the basis of objective evidence, and this means that knowledge that is gained subjectively must be checked to see that it supported by evidence.

EBP, a key concept in modern health care, is one element of clinical governance (DOH 1999), a framework for the continual improvement of services and quality in the NHS, the purpose of which is to ensure that clinical decisions are based on the most up-to-date evidence and that clear national standards are set to reduce local variations in access to and outcomes of health care. Clinical governance has the following key elements:

- To set national standards for health services through development of national service frameworks and the National Institute for Clinical Excellence (NICE).
- To provide mechanisms for assessing local delivery of high-quality services, reinforced by a new statutory duty to quality.
- To provide support for life-long learning.
- To develop effective systems for monitoring the delivery of quality standards in the form of the Commission for Health Improvement, the NHS Performance Framework and surveys of patient/user experience (DOH 1999).

All health professionals are accountable for their individual practice and are responsible for making sure that their knowledge and skills are current. This implies that any care given is based on the most up-to-date knowledge available.

EBP forms an essential element in the quality of health care and is directly related to clinical care in that clinically effective practice is based on national standards, frameworks and research.

A systematic approach to acquiring evidence

Systematic acquisition of evidence provides the information from which standards and protocols for care are developed. Standards and protocols related to the provision of care are written by employers to guide the process of care. Health trusts use national guidelines based on the work of the National

Institute for Clinical Excellence (NICE) and evidence from research as the basis for protocols. Each employee has a duty to keep up-to-date with, and refer to, guidelines that are supplied by their employer to inform their specific area of care, and to work to protocols.

Research is the means of gathering evidence, and thus the source of guidelines and protocols. Nurses should have a working knowledge of the research process to enable them to appraise and understand the evidence that is presented as the basis for care, and be able to make a judgement on validity.

McInness *et al.* (2001) suggest that evidence is not easily integrated into practice. The reasons that they offer for this are that research literature can be poorly organised and not easy to read, making it particularly hard for busy practitioners to access. The same authors also acknowledge the poor quality of some research. These comments make it clear that evidence is not always easy to access/understand, neither is it always sound. Health professionals must be able to interpret the information that is given to them to enable them to question evidence when it is unclear or unconvincing. The application of EBP lies with each health professional who must exercise judgement about the applicability of knowledge, whether it is evidence-based or subjective. Senior members of the team should have sufficient knowledge to support less experienced nurses, but all registered nurses should have a working knowledge that equips them to question the soundness of practice.

A part of professional life must be the acquisition of knowledge that informs patient/client care. Access to information through electronic journals and websites makes information readily accessible. Most health trusts have access points for internet searches and this makes it so much easier for nurses to keep informed and current in their practice.

Evidence–based care or patient preference?

There may be some instances where a treatment or practice, even though based on evidence, may not be appropriate for a patient. Thought and consideration are required to be given by practitioners at each care intervention. This makes the argument for evidence-based practice turn on itself. You may reasonably ask why objective evidence cannot be applied in all cases when it is likely to be effective. The response to this rests in the nature of health care practice, which is described by McCormack *et al.* (2002) as practice that takes place in a variety of settings, communities and cultures. To add to this complexity, there are other relevant influences, for example psychosocial and economic factors. Taking all these factors into account it is reasonable to assume that thought needs to be given to the application of practice. While practice should be based on evidence, it is also important to establish that the patient is suited to this care, and willing to accept the proposed treatment.

Informed decisions and patient choice

One example of advocated treatment being found unacceptable to the patient, would arise in the case of a family who do not wish to have their child vaccinated with the triple measles, mumps and rubella (MMR) vaccine. The family might hold strong views about the safety of triple vaccine. Here the parents' wishes might conflict with those of professionals, who have convincing reasons why children should be protected from childhood infections. There are no easy answers to this type of problem, and decisions taken must be carefully considered in the light of evidence that is presented from a range of sources. The patients', or in this case the parents', wishes are vital. When decisions about care are to be made the nurse's role is to provide information that can enable the patient to make an informed decision, but in the end the choice rests with the patient.

Planning decisions about care are normally considered by the care team, and a long-term treatment plan, though initially developed by one nurse, would not rest with a single individual. The plan would be discussed by the team to ensure that it was suitable and allow all team members to understand the goals and process of care. Daily evaluation of circumstances would, however, rest with an individual and would rely on informed decision making.

> **Example**
>
> In the case of your patient, can you deduce any reason why a proposed treatment that is known to be based on the best available evidence may not be suitable?

Professional practice relies on nurses being competent in a range of specified outcomes (UKCC 2001), successful achievement of which equips nurses to practice. Practice requires that decisions are made, and that implies that each professional should be knowledgeable in their subject area and have the ability to translate their knowledge to support practice. Knowledge in itself has only limited value if it is used without due consideration of the effect that it might have on a situation. Thus a key aspect of professional practice is the ability to interpret and apply knowledge in widely varying circumstances. It is around the varying circumstances that decisions must be made that assure that care is appropriate and each nurse is accountable for the decisions that they make about patient care (NMC 2002).

LEARNING THROUGH REFLECTION

Many of the issues raised in this chapter illustrate the complexity of nursing practice and demonstrate how thinking skills and decision making are essential to good practice. Not only is nursing practice complex it is also dynamic, and changes with developments in health policy and scientific knowledge. For nurses this means that every patient contact is unique and that over a period of time a great deal of experience is generated from nursing practice. Nursing practice, taken in its widest sense, means working with other health and social care practitioners to provide the assessment, organisation and management of holistic care for patients.

Reflection is a great way to learn. It enables nurses to capitalise on what they do well and see how to improve the aspects of care that did not go so well. Taylor (2000) stresses this by stating how the unconsidered life is transformed, through the process of reflection, into one that is consciously aware, self-potentiating and purposeful. All recently qualified nurses will have been taught to use reflection as a method of learning, for just as EBP is a key concept in current nursing practice, so is reflection. Reflection has particular value to learning in nursing because of the richness of experience in practice and the direct observation that nurses are able to make about how the care that they and the health care team give affects patients.

Reflection and practice

Reflection can and should take place during the process of practice. Schon (1983) refers to this as 'reflection in action'. It also takes place after the event, which Schon refers to as 'reflection on action'. Sometimes reflection is private, at other times it is shared with colleagues or may even form part of a team meeting.

> **Example**
>
> Think about your chosen patient, and reflect on one aspect of care that you feel pleased with. Identify what was good about this particular aspect of care and why it was good. Also make a list of the 'good' parts that could be transferred to benefit the care of future patients.

The exercise that you have undertaken is an illustration of reflecting on practice, learning from it and using the learning to inform and develop future practice. This is why reflection is so beneficial in nursing. In part it is explained because of the uniqueness of each situation demands new thinking and reasoning and this accumulates over time as experience increases.

Reflecting on action is a deliberate event. It can be a very effective learning experience for the individual nurse or for the team. Each nurse should regularly take time to reflect on their practice, considering their knowledge and skills, the evidence base from which care is given and the many influences that impinge on care.

Group reflection probably occurs informally in many teams at hand-over meetings when care is discussed. Reflection by the team in a more formal sense provides opportunity for review of patient care on a planned and regular basis. Like the individual nurse, the care team considers their knowledge and skills, the evidence base from which care is given, the influences on care, that are raised in models of nursing, and take a general reflective view of the care provided for each patient. Group thinking can be productive, with each member contributing an individual perspective, and everyone learning from the others in the group. Shaw (1981) suggests that groups make better-quality decisions than individuals, which has particular significance when so much is at stake for patients. However, some caution needs to be exercised when a group reflects, on account of a phenomenon known as groupthink, whereby pressures for conformity and for keeping within the boundaries of accepted practice stifle creative thinking (Robbins 1986).

Learning often occurs when something happens that is disappointing or does not turn out the right way. It is this type of experience that most frequently makes people think about what they have or have not done and how it could have been more effectively achieved. It is not enough only to reflect and recognise where things went wrong: that is evaluation of the incident. Reflection is more than evaluation – it involves new learning. For learning to occur it is first necessary to identify what, in the case of a negative experience, went wrong. It is then essential to take the necessary steps to remedy the deficit and put it right. It may be as simple as recognising that work has been done without sufficient thought and that corners have been cut. In this instance the practitioner knows what should be done but has failed to do it correctly. The learning will be in the nature of accepting that however great the pressures, sufficient time must be given to each patient and procedure. It may, however, be that new learning needs to take place, perhaps a new skill needs to be learned, maybe from a colleague who has the necessary expertise. Sometimes knowledge is out of date and must be updated by reading or by attending study days. Very often in primary care nurses come across health problems that are new to them and they have to find the information that is needed to enable them to provide effective care. As you can see, learning involves taking some action. The purpose of reflective practice is to actively enable learning so

that it becomes integral to routine practice. If a nurse constantly reflects on practice, learns from it and changes practice in response to learning, practice will not become static and out of date.

Aids to reflection

A number of frameworks have been designed to help the process of reflection. Many nurses are introduced to reflection by using the staged process advocated by Gibbs (1988). Gibbs's model offers a cycle to guide nurses through the reflective process:

- describe what happened
- explore the thoughts and feelings that occurred as part of the experience
- evaluate what was good and bad about the experience
- analyse the experience in order to better understand it
- consider what else could have been done, and finally
- make an action plan to determine how the situation would be handled should it occur again.

This cycle of steps gives an easy-to-follow process, guiding the nurse through reflection. There are other frameworks that facilitate the reflective process, for example Burnard (1991), Boud, Keogh and Walker (1985) and Goodman (1984). Goodman's approach focuses on levels of reflection, suggesting three levels of increasing complexity. The first level consists of a simple approach that involves considering how the job was done with regard to technical efficiency and effectiveness, and in terms of accountability. The second level takes a wider view, looking at the implications and consequences of the nurse's actions and beliefs, which includes the underlying rationale for practice. The third, most complex, level draws on all the considerations in levels one and two, and adds ethical and political considerations and developments.

There are distinct differences between the approaches that are taken by Gibbs and Goodman. Gibbs offers a framework to facilitate structured thinking while Goodman pushes the boundaries of thinking to levels of considerable complexity. Examination of different approaches helps nurses to choose the one most suited to the situation. As with models of nursing the most suitable approach to reflection may vary with differing experiences and so it is beneficial to have a range of approaches to draw upon.

CONCLUSION

This chapter has covered some of the key factors that influence and inform professional practice in nursing. This should create awareness of sources of nursing knowledge and reinforce earlier learning that introduced the nature and purpose of nursing models. There is no doubt that practice is complex and nurses can only truly attempt to meet the needs of patients if they are able to understand and manage complexity. The value of models of nursing is that, in representing the complex nature of practice, they act as prompts. Because each model is presented in diagrammatic form it enables the same detailed process of assessment, planning, implementation and evaluation to take place for every patient. Professional skill comes into play as infinitely variable information is analysed and interpreted into personal and individual plans of care that take account of very differing needs. The skill of the nurse is needed to manage patient information and translate it, with the patient's collaboration, into meaningful and appropriate delivery of care. Nurses must therefore be knowledgeable and skilful. The dynamic nature of health care means that new knowledge is constantly emerging, and health practitioners are obliged to keep up to date with the latest developments.

Knowledge and the validity of information are requirements for planning effective, economic care. Quality in care is high on the government agenda for improving the National Health Service (DOH 2000). Receiving care that is based on objective information is an essential part of provision; application of care without thought or consideration of the individuality of people would go against the ethos of professional practice (Norman and Cowley 1999). Norman and Cowley state that knowledge based on evidence is valuable and should underpin protocols and guidelines. Information that is collated and current greatly assists practitioners. Blind acceptance of evidence is not, however, consistent with professional practice, one criterion of which is autonomy. Reflective practitioners who are constantly learning on the job are fundamental to the profession – nurses who can plan appropriate care on an individual basis, with the patient, and are able to be justify their decisions.

REFERENCES

Aggleton, P. and Chalmers, A. (2000) *Nursing Models and Nursing Practice* (2nd edn). London: Macmillan.

Boud, D., Keogh, R. and Walker, D. (1985) *Reflections: Turning Experience into Learning.* London: Kogan Page.

Burnard, P. (1991) Improving through reflection. *Journal of District Nursing,* May:10–12.

Carey, R.G. and Posovac, E.J. (1982) Using patient information to identify areas for service improvement. *HMC Review,* 7(2): 42–8.

Department of Health (1999) *Clinical Governance: Quality in the New NHS.* London: DOH.

Department of Health (2000) *The NHS Plan: A Plan for Investment, A Plan for Reform.* London: The Stationery Office.

Fawcett, J. (1984) *Analysis and Evaluation of Conceptual Models of Nursing.* Philadelphia, PA: F.A. Davis.

Gibbs, G. (1988) *Learning by Doing: A Guide to Teaching and Learning Methods.* Oxford: Oxford Polytechnic Further Education Unit.

Gibbs, G. (1997) *Improving Student Learning: Theory and Practice.* Oxford: Oxford Brookes University, Centre for Staff and Learning Development.

Goodman, J. (1984) Reflection and teacher education: a case study and theoretical analysis. *Interchange,* 15(3): 19–26.

Henderson, V. (1966) *The Nature of Nursing.* London: Collier Macmillan.

McCormack, B., Kitson, A., Harvey, G., Rycroft-Malone, J., Titchen, A. and Seers, K. (2002) Getting evidence into practice: the meaning of context. *Journal of Advanced Nursing,* 38(1): 94–104.

McInness, E., Harvey, G., Duff, L., Fennessy, G., Seers, K. and Clark, E. (2001) Implementing evidence-based practice in clinical situations. *Nursing Standard,* 15: 40–4.

Neuman, B. (ed.) (1989) *The Neuman Systems Model.* Norwalk, OH: Appleton & Lange.

Norman, I. and Cowley, S. (eds) (1999) *The Changing Nature of Nursing.* Oxford: Blackwell Science.

Nursing and Midwifery Council (2002) *Code of Professional Conduct.* London: NMC.

Orem, D.E. (1980) *Nursing: Concepts of Practice.* New York: McGraw Hill.

Pearson, A., Vaughn, B. and Fitzgerald, M. (1996) *Models for Nursing Practice* (2nd edn). Oxford: Butterworth–Heinemann.

Peplau, H.E. (1988) *Interpersonal Relations in Nursing*. Basingstoke: Macmillan Education.

Riehl, J. and Roy, C. (eds) (1980) *Conceptual Models for Nursing Practice* (2nd edn). Norwalk, CT: Appleton-Century-Crofts.

Robbins, S.P. (1986) *Organisational Behaviour: Concepts, Controversies and Applications* (3rd edn). Englewood Cliffs, NJ: Prentice Hall.

Roper, N., Logan, W.W. and Tierney, A.J. (1980) *The Elements of Nursing*. Edinburgh: Churchill Livingstone.

Roper, N., Logan, W.W. and Tierney, A.J. (2000) *Roper–Logan–Tierney Model of Nursing: The Activities of Living Model*. Edinburgh: Churchill Livingstone.

Roy, C. (1976) *Introduction to Nursing: An Adaptation Model*. Englewood Cliffs, NJ: Prentice Hall.

Schon, D. (1983) *The Reflective Practitioner*. New York: Basic Books.

Shaw, M.E. (1981) *Group Dynamics* (3rd edn). New York: McGraw-Hill.

Taylor, B.J. (2000) *Reflective Practice: A Guide for Nurses and Midwives*. Buckingham: Open University.

UK Central Council for Nursing, Midwifery and Health Visiting (2001) *Fitness for Practice and Purpose*. London: UKCC.

Wells, J.S.G. (1999) The growth of managerialism and its impact on nursing and the NHS. In I. Norman and S. Cowley (eds), *The Changing Nature of Nursing*. Oxford: Blackwell Science.

Yura, H. and Walsh, M. (1967) *The Nursing Process*. Norwalk, CT: Appleton-Century-Crofts.

8

Professional issues in community nursing

Jenny Parry and Judith Parsons

Learning outcomes

- Identify the use of professional approaches in community nursing practice.
- Analyse the similarities and differences between hospital and community nursing.
- Recognise the complex nature of decision making within a community setting.
- Discuss contemporary innovations in community nursing practice.

INTRODUCTION

This chapter will examine the professional issues that impact on the nurse working in the community. Many of the skills that a nurse uses in an acute setting are transferable to community nursing, but the focus of the work tends to be different, because it relates to people in their everyday lives, either in their own homes, general practice, school, work, clinic or other familiar environments. Some of the skills acquired previously in the acute setting are transferable, but there is a need to develop new approaches and additional knowledge in order to function efficiently and effectively.

WHAT ARE PROFESSIONAL APPROACHES TO CARE?

Nursing practice in the United Kingdom (UK) is currently regulated by the Nursing and Midwifery Council (NMC). The nurse has responsibilities within these regulations towards clients, the public, the profession, the employer and to themselves.

In the community the nurse is potentially responsible to a wider spectrum of clients and professionals on a day to day basis. They are a diverse group of people because of the range of client groups, professionals and voluntary agencies with whom she may come into contact. Legislation may also impact upon the role; for example: the Mental Health Act 1983, the Children Act 1989, and the Human Rights Act 1998. Nursing practice in the community differs from that in the hospital, in that it is not necessarily observable by another professional, but is often only seen by clients, their family and informal carers. This gives more autonomy to the community nurse but places more responsibility on them, which will require them to develop sophisticated decision making skills. The extent to which this takes place will be affected by job descriptions, clinical grade and expectations and the requirements of the nursing team and the trust/employer.

One area of community nursing practice where staff nurses may find significant differences between hospital and community nursing is in the approach to the assessment of clients and families. This is closely linked to the standards for community specialist practice (UKCC 1994). This may mean that some staff nurses will not be undertaking initial assessments of clients or families as they would have done routinely in hospital. Role activities will vary considerably between different disciplines of community nursing and areas within the UK. An example of this might be a staff nurse working in a health visiting team who could be undertaking routine child development work related to assessment and screening, whilst a staff nurse in a district nursing team may not be undertaking any initial assessment work. It is vital that all levels of staff in this environment, where the clients are not monitored in the same way as on a hospital ward, carry out continuous assessment. This demonstrates how closely the role of the community staff nurse is associated with that of the specialist practitioner and the way in which teams function (Vanclay 1998). It is discussed in more detail in Chapter 6. These different approaches to care can be explored more closely from a professional perspective, as in the past roles were very clearly defined and supported by legislation. This meant for example that the core activities associated with particularly health visiting could only be carried out by registered health visitors (Nurses, Midwives and Health Visitors Act 1979). As health care demands have become more complex and sophisticated new roles have evolved, such as that of the nurse consultant, whilst the role of community specialist practitioners continues to develop and change with staff nurses being integral to this policy (DOH 1999a, 2000a, 2002a). Thus there is a need to define clearly the essential requirements of any community nursing service (Audit Commission 1999), and at the time of writing many changes are taking place (DOH 2002a.).

KNOWING WHAT YOU ARE DOING

All nurses come to community nursing bringing the skills and knowledge that they have used in the acute setting (Canham and Moore 2002). In the acute working environment, when the nurse has uncertainties there are other members of the team nearby to call upon. Usually knowledge and clinical skills that are used within a familiar environment will enable the nurse to be confident and competent in her nursing interventions. It is important for any

nurse working in a new environment to recognise the skills that they bring with them. These can continue to be used and are known as transferable skills. It is equally important for nurses in a new setting to identify the new skills they may need to acquire. These can be obtained in different ways and there are a number of resources that the nurse can draw on:

- *The senior nurse/line manager* will be a resource for relevant policies and protocols, and could be the relevant person to assist staff in identifying the areas of practice that need further development. They may be in a position to enable staff to access appropriate study days and short courses to facilitate continuing professional development.
- *Clinical supervision* is increasingly available. It should provide the opportunity for staff to explore and develop best practice within a safe environment (Butterworth *et al.* 1998).
- *Code of Professional Conduct* (NMC 2002) is a useful aid to check the standards that are required.
- *The individual approach* can be to use the SWOT analysis (Hannagan 2000), which enables the nurse to identify opportunities and threats or, more simply, to list strengths and weaknesses.
- *The use of reflection* can aid all of the above activities, but can be particularly useful in helping to identify areas of practice that have worked well and find ways of approaching other areas where further professional development is required (Johns 1995). Reflection is explored in greater detail in Chapter 7.

Exercise

It would be useful if you firstly reviewed your actual/potential professional responsibilities in the community nursing environment. Consider the setting in which you meet clients – home, clinic, health centre, GP surgery, workplace.

Reflect on and list the key differences you find practising in this setting. Using the information on key differences, list your transferable skills and those that may need further development. List the new knowledge and skills that you need to acquire.

Some of the points identified could include issues surrounding the need not only to transfer and adapt skills, but also to provide care in a flexible and innovative way. Professional competence is a complex set of knowledge and skills, which integrates knowledge, judgement, reasoning, personal qualities, skills, values and beliefs. This means that the transference of skills and knowledge may need to be interpreted in a more flexible manner, where the environment or situation is less clinical than has been worked in previously, as would be the case, for example, in a refugee centre, where there is little understanding of the UK health care system and therefore the client expectations are different.

This may often mean adapting to the needs of the client and responding in a more holistic manner to their needs than might have occurred in a hospital environment. The nurse's response will be concerned with information giving to enable the clients to understand the differences in the UK health and welfare system. Working as a community nurse means starting out as a novice in this new setting but very quickly transferring and adapting existing skills and acquiring new ones so as to develop into a competent and ultimately proficient practitioner (Benner 1984).

A useful exercise is to observe the senior nurse who is accountable for the caseload or client group and identify the different ways in which they interact with clients and respond to needs (McIntosh 1996). Experienced and skilled nurses will practise with confidence and competence and provide a flexible and innovative service, and they can be considered expert nurses (Benner 1984). This level of expert practice, which draws on their experience, education and evidence, is often called professional artistry (Schon 1991).

Whilst staff nurses or student nurses cannot be expected to work at this level there are several important points associated with this way of practising. These expert practitioners are comfortable within their roles and with time, experience and education staff nurses can be expected to use some of the same skills within their own practice. The extent to which these can be developed may depend on employers. It is also important to remember that staff nurses are normally part of a team, and whilst not fulfilling the same role as the community specialist practitioner (UKCC 1994), will complement the service offered to the clients. Nursing in this context requires a practitioner who is able to maintain safe high standards of practice and be flexible and innovative. These can be seen to be centred around the set of core skills listed below:

- assessment of individuals, families and carers
- decision making
- clinical expertise
- patient/client teaching
- public health and health promotion
- interest in and respect for the client community
- effective communication skills, underpinning all of the above.

These core skills recognise that practice takes place in a real-life setting (Carr 2001) rather than the more focused acute sector of care. Nursing in the community is multi-faceted, encompassing diverse client needs. The power normally lies with the client rather than the nurse. This is because clients potentially have more control over care when receiving health services either in their own home or in other familiar environments, such as their workplace or GP premises. They usually feel more comfortable and are not normally functioning within the sick role (Parsons 1951).

DECISION MAKING

This should be based on information gathered mainly from the initial assessment and from ongoing contact with the patient/family. It is not just about interpreting medical diagnosis or clinical interventions, but taking the patient's real life agenda into account. Decision making is influenced by many factors that can be seen to inter-relate, which increases the complexity of the task (see Figure 8.1).

These factors may have different emphases according to the practice area, but all can be found in community nursing. They are evident in the following example.

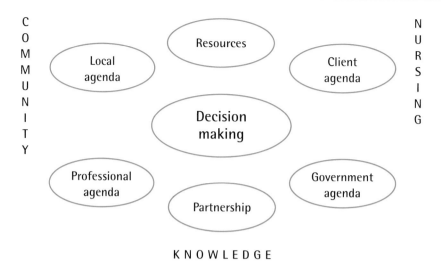

Figure 8.1 *Decision making in community nursing*

Example

Wayne, aged 13 years, has been truanting. He turns up at a confidential drop-in session that the school nurse runs. In conversation he tells her that he looks after his mother, who has multiple sclerosis, and that this is the reason for his absences. He adds that his mother is entirely dependent on him for most of her care needs.

The factors the school nurse will need to consider include:

- the needs of the child
- the mother–son relationship
- client agenda – who is the client in this situation?
- confidentiality
- her knowledge of child carers
- the government agenda re truancy and care in the community
- the law
- partnership working
- available resources for this family's needs.

When trying to make decisions in such a situation a holistic assessment needs to be undertaken. Any

nurse working in the community may have some of the knowledge required to work with this family, but how they prioritise the different factors will depend on their experience and branch of nursing. It is likely that more information is going to be required about Wayne and his mother, such as the family and its membership and whether any other professionals are already involved.

Exercise

Can you think of any other information you would like if you were a member of the school nursing team looking at Wayne's case?

Figure 8.1 demonstrates how the nurse assessing care can ensure the wider context of community nursing is addressed. This contrasts with nursing in an acute care setting, where the patient may be seen in the more limited context of daily living needs. In community nursing, decisions cannot be made in isolation from the client's real-life situation (Carr 2001), which reinforces the government's agenda on working in partnership and empowering people (DOH 1998, 2000a). The client is central to any care decisions that are to be made and should be consulted about what their goals are for any intervention by health and social care professionals or voluntary agencies, so that a collaborative care package can be developed (DOH 2002a).

As suggested by Figure 8.1, there are various factors that need to be considered. When undertaking this process the nurse must be skilled in needs assessment, goal setting, intervention and evaluating outcomes (Southard *et al.* 1994). The nurse should examine the factors in each individual client situation and consider the possible course of action and potential outcomes. This will enable them to anticipate any unintended consequences that may impact on the family, carers, group or community. The challenge to any assessing nurse is to find a mutual understanding of the needs of their client and attempt to meet them while taking into account the local availability of resources. There are studies in mental health using decision trees (Concoran 1986). This approach has been found by Bonner (2001) to be time-consuming and complex, but the ideology of having alternative partnerships of care can be utilised by the community nurse to ensure that all factors have been considered. The use of the decision-making diagram in Figure 8.1 provides an aid to assessment that is simpler to use. The client is central to the decision making, and by ensuring that each factor has been addressed all needs can potentially be met. A staff nurse may already have gained some knowledge of the client's situation, either through hand-over, medical records, referral information, or previous assessment. These are all cues to identifying the real-life situation for the client and their family (Carr 2001). They can be drawn upon to contribute to the decision making of potential intervention activities, which may be required to meet their needs (Buckingham 2000). Benner *et al.* (1996) recognise how these cues shape decisions in relating them to previous knowledge.

Example

A client presents for a routine cervical smear screening. On discussion with the practice nurse she states that she is 'passing water a lot' and seems very thirsty. Interpreting these clues, the practice nurse would undertake basic investigations for diabetes.

Nurses use previous knowledge and experience to support their decision making (Benner 1984). Clinical supervision can support nurses in their decisions, reinforcing quality of care through reflection and can also enable them to identify deficits in their knowledge base for professional development (Butterworth *et al.* 1998).

The notion of concordance, that is negotiation between health care professionals and the patient/client and family, is central to community nursing. It is concerned with giving full information and establishing a contract of care with the patient (Alder 1999). This can be achieved with effective interpersonal skills, collaboration and consent within a patient-centred approach. The nurse will need good understanding of client health beliefs and and awareness of the barriers to communication that can lead to ineffective collaboration in care.

The locality in which people live and work will have identified resources that may meet the needs of the client group. The knowledge of these resources can be accessed from a range of sources: community specialist practitioners, primary care and health and social care trusts or their equivalents, local libraries, citizens advice bureaux, voluntary agencies and the internet. Part of the way that community nurses can become familiar with local resources and needs is through health needs assessment and use of the community profile, which has been written about in Chapter 3 (see also Robinson and Elkan 1996; Worth 1996; Billings and Cowley 1995).

CURRENT INNOVATIONS IN PRACTICE

Amongst the current innovations in practice is the use of nurse prescribing to complement and provide more holistic client care. It can be seen as one of the major changes that have occurred in nursing. The concept was first developed in community nursing as a response to the Cumberlege Report, which identified the need in 1986 (DHSS 1986).

The Medicinal Products Prescription by Nurses etc. Act 1992 gave district nurses and health visitors independent prescribing powers from a limited formulary. This group of specialist nurses, which includes any practice nurse with either of these qualifications, has been trained since 1999. Nurse prescribing education is now within the qualifying degree programme for the health visitor and district nurse specialities. The *Review of Prescribing, Supply and Administration of Medicines* (DOH 1999a) suggested that prescribing powers might be extended to more nurses and after a 3-month consultation with professional organisations, ministers announced in May 2001 that nurse prescribing would be extended to more nurses and to a wider range of medicines. The *Nurse Prescribing Extended Formulary* (BMA and Royal Pharmaceutical Society of Great Britain 2002) has increased the prescription-only medicines intended for nursing care in four main areas; minor injuries; minor ailments; health promotion/maintenance and palliative care. The formulary includes all General Sales List (GSL), the so-called over the counter medicines, and pharmacy-only (P) medicines.

The *Review of Prescribing* (DOH 1999a) recommended two types of prescriber:

- The independent prescriber, who is responsible for the assessment of patients with undiagnosed conditions and for the clinical management, which may include prescribing.
- The dependent prescriber, who is reponsible for the continuing care of patients who have been clinically assessed by an independent prescriber (doctor or dentist). This continuing care may include prescribing from individual clinical management plans. It was also proposed that pharmacists and other allied health care professionals would also become dependent prescribers (now referred to as supplementary prescribers).

Supplementary prescribing has now become part of the extended nurse-independent prescribing course. Supplementary prescribing will enable the nurses and pharmacists to continue treatment regimes within an agreed plan, prescribing from most areas of the British national formulary. Scotland, Wales and Northern Ireland at the time of writing are to decide whether and when it will be implemented in their countries.

Supplementary prescribing is intended to provide patients with a quicker and more efficient access to medication (DOH 2003). The aim is for more nurses and other allied professions to prescribe and is based on the intention to enhance patient/client care by providing continuity and using health professional skills to their best effect.

Prescribing is a team activity in as much as the independent prescriber utilises the knowledge and expertise of all team members to enable and support their prescribing decisions. This supports partnership working between health professionals and gives a greater understanding of roles, responsibilities and accountability in patient care (Basford and Bowskill 2002).

The increase in prescribing powers has led to nurses taking a leading role in introducing new services, such as nurse-led minor ailments clinics, and chronic disease management could be nurse- or pharamacist-led. This could be an area of care in which staff nurses in the future may be required to develop knowledge and skills.

FUTURE CHANGES IN PRACTICE

Since 1997, when the Labour party returned to government, there have been many new approaches to the NHS, not least focusing on a primary care-led service (DOH 1997). These changes are detailed more fully in social policy textbooks, but their cumulative impact is evident in *The NHS Plan* (DOH 2000a), a 10-year project for the delivery of health care in England. This document summarises government health strategy, providing an umbrella approach to recent policies based on the modernisation agenda for health. Subsequent papers (DOH 2001a, 2002b) detail the ways in which the NHS plan is to be implemented in primary care. The new strategies have had an impact on community nursing and the ways in which nurses are expected to provide health care (DOH 1999b, 2002a). Other countries in the UK are at different stages of planning at the time of writing, but either have produced (Scottish Executive Health Department 2000), or can be expected to produce similar documents to meet the needs of health and social care delivery within Scotland, Wales and Northern Ireland.

One of the most important changes that is taking place is the move towards a public health agenda throughout all the countries of the UK. This degree of focus on public health has not been seen since the 19th century. It was in that period and in response to that public health agenda that health visiting, occupational health nursing, district nursing and school nursing first developed. So now existing community nursing services will have to adapt, and perhaps in some cases re-invent themselves, in order to meet the public health demands of the 21st century. The Department of Health for England has identified new approaches to providing care, and new ways of working (DOH 2000a). They include not only a public health and health promotion role for all nurses, but an emphasis on more effective assessment and delivery of care, chronic disease management and the implementation of the national service frameworks (NSFs). Resource packs have been developed for health visiting and school nursing to help to facilitate staff in these new ways of working (DOH 2001b, 2001c). A range of strategies is being put in place by primary care and health and social care trusts to enable these new policy initiatives to be implemented. In the other countries in the UK similar initiatives are being adopted, particularly in Scotland (Scottish Executive Health Department 2001). This means that all nurses working in the community will be required to take on some of this new work, such as providing more acute care at home and managing the care of patients with a range of chronic diseases. Specialist practitioners will be delivering some of these innovations in care, together with staff nurses in their teams. In other instances staff nurses will be taking on new roles, enabling the specialist practitioners to work in other ways. These developments enable community nursing to develop practice in new and more flexible and innovative ways. *Liberating the Talents* (DOH 2002a) cites examples from around England of how all levels of community nurses can be supported in working in new ways. In Scotland, in order to meet the health needs of the population, the Health Department of the Scottish Executive have found new ways for nurses to deliver the public health agenda (Scottish Executive Health Department 2001).

All community nursing staff will find themselves working to deliver the modernisation agenda. One of the ways this will take place in England is through the standards set by the NSFs. To date the

following have been published for: mental health (DOH 1999c), coronary heart disease (DOH 2000b), cancer (2000c), older people (2001e), and diabetes (DOH 2001f). The NSF for children is awaiting publication. The NSFs have been put in place to ensure quality and equity of care. They provide standards for care of the various groups and are concerned with health care delivery in both the acute and primary care sectors. Some, such as the ones for mental health and older people, very specifically require collaboration with other agencies. A good example of this is the single assessment process highlighted in the NSF for older people (DOH 2001e). This process will place the patient at the centre of the assessment process, which will only take place once, no matter how many health and social care professionals are involved. So community nurses may find themselves relying on an assessment carried out by a care manager. The importance of respecting one another's professional expertise and experience will be very significant in this process (Ovretveit 1997). It will prevent clients undergoing repeated assessments and suffering from assessment fatigue.

Other examples of flexible ways of delivering health care to the population can be seen by the way in which the government has set up initiatives such as NHS Direct. This 24-hour telephone help line is staffed by specially trained nurses. It has proved popular with the public (O'Cathain et al. 2000), but initially received less favourable reviews from doctors, who were concerned about the quality of the service (Hayes 2000). Recent signs suggest that some of these initial misgivings may have been resolved and that the service is now being more accepted (Sadler 2002). Another initiative is the use of telephone triage in general practice, which is used to screen clients and decide who can best meet their needs (Richards and Tawfik 2000). These services are normally undertaken by nurse practitioners or practice nurses who have undertaken additional education. It is likely that this type of work will continue to increase and community nurses are in key positions to take this forward.

One of the other areas of innovation where nurses are at the forefront of service delivery is walk-in centres. These have been established in accessible localities for local communities to offer flexible health care (DOH 2002a). They are normally staffed by a team of nurses led by an experienced senior nurse, who is frequently a nurse practitioner or a community specialist practitioner in practice nursing. All these initiatives are team based and will require a level of skill mix in order to deliver them efficiently and effectively.

In order to deliver these innovations in practice there will have to be effective leadership from senior nurses. Research has shown that some of the most effective leaders are those who are found to possess emotional intelligence. They rise to the top of organisations (Goleman 1998). These skills may be summed up as people skills used in a management context. Corning (2002) has shown how skills such as employee development, teamwork, negotiation, self management, and decision making enable effective leadership. She also adds other characteristics such as futuristic thinking, empathy and interpersonal skills. When taken in context with the way in which care delivery is changing in community nursing these can be seen to be very desirable qualities for senior nurses to possess.

Emotional intelligence is associated with transformational leadership, which is the way in which futuristic thinking can be developed. These attributes can be applied to change management and Hill (2002) considers that there are certain factors that need to be taken into account, for example the importance of generating energy.

Exercise

Think about the senior nurses or managers who have inspired you. What did you like about their leadership style?

It is important for senior nurses to have the energy to take the vision for the future of community nursing forward. This can sometimes be difficult if staff feel threatened and demoralised by constant change and teams are reluctant to co-operate with new ways of working. This is when transformational leaders are needed to enable team members to share in the vision for the future and facilitate staff in implementing change. Leaders will be required to develop new ways of thinking about issues and problems, and to be very creative and innovative, whilst also motivating their teams. At the same time change will have to take place within the constraints of the organisation, in this case the NHS. Hill (2002) indicates that it is important to set structures in place to allow change to take place. Currently, this is provided by the various health departments in the four countries of the UK.

CONCLUSION

Professional approaches to care in community nursing can be identified by the need to be competent and confident in settings that do not normally provide the same level of immediate support to the nurse that is available within an acute setting. This means that the nurse is required to develop a range of skills that will enable her to professionally practise with confidence, establishing an environment of partnership with patients in a real-life situation. Some of these skills will have been acquired in the acute setting, whilst others will be developed when working in community nursing. Assessment undertaken in the community looks at the wider picture (see Figure 8.1) which entails greater complexity in decision making. Current innovations in the health and social care agenda will mean that all nurses will be required to adapt and be flexible and open to change.

FURTHER READING

Bishop, V. and Scott, I. (2001) Developing clinical practice. In *Challenges in Clinical Practice: Professional Developments in Nursing*. (2nd edn). Basingstoke: Palgrave.

Johns, C. (2000) *Becoming a Reflective Practitioner*. Oxford: Blackwell Science.

REFERENCES

Alder, B. (1999) *Psychology of Health: Applications of Psychology for Health Professionals* (2nd edn). Singapore: Harwood Academic Publishers.

Audit Commission (1999) *First Assessment: A Review of District Nursing Services in England and Wales*. London: Audit Commission for Local Authorities and the NHS in England and Wales.

Basford, L. and Bowskill, D. (2002) Celebrating the present, challenging the future of nurse prescribing. In *Topics in Nurse Prescribing* (*British Journal of Community Nursing* monograph). Wiltshire: Mark Allen Publishers.

Benner, P. (1984) *From Novice to Expert: Excellence and Power in Clinical Nursing Practice*. Boston, MA: Addison-Wesley.

Benner, P., Tanner, C. and Chesla, C. (1996) *Expertise in Nursing Practice: Caring, Clinical Judgment and Ethics*. New York: Springer.

Billings, J.R. and Cowley, S. (1995) Approaches to community needs assessment: a literature review. *Journal of Advanced Nursing*, 22(4): 721–30.

Bonner, G. (2001) Decision making for health care professionals: use of decision trees within the community mental setting. *Journal of Advanced Nursing*, 35(3): 349–56.

British Medical Association and Royal Pharmaceutical Society of Great Britain (2002) *Nurse Prescribing Formulary (2002–3)*. London: BMA and RPSGB.

Buckingham, C. and Adams, A. (2000) Classifying clinical decision making: interpreting nursing intuition, heuristics and medical diagnosis. *Journal of Advanced Nursing*, 32(4): 990–8.

Butterworth, T., Faugier, J. and Burnard, P. (1998) *Clinical Supervision and Mentorship in Nursing* (2nd edn). Cheltenham: Stanley Thornes.

Canham, J. and Moore, S. (2002) Learning approaches in the practice context. In J. Canham and J. Bennett (eds), *Mentorship in Community Nursing: Challenges and Opportunities*. Oxford: Blackwell Science.

Carr, S. (2001) Nursing in the community – impact on the practice agenda. *Journal of Clinical Nursing*, 10(3): 330–6.

Children Act (1989) London: HMSO.

Concoran, S. (1986) Decision analysis: a step-by-step guide for making clinical decisions. *Nursing and Health Care*, 7.

Corning, S. (2002) Profiling and developing nurse leaders. *Journal of Nursing Administration*, 32(7/8): 373–5.

Department of Health (1997) *The New NHS: Modern, Dependable*. London: The Stationery Office.

Department of Health (1998) *Working in Partnership*. London: The Stationery Office.

Department of Health (1999a) *Review of Prescribing, Supply and Administration of Medicines* (Final Report). London: The Stationery Office.

Department of Health (1999b) *Making a Difference*. London: The Stationery Office.

Department of Health (1999c) *National Service Framework for Mental Health*. London: The Stationery Office.

Department of Health (2000a) *The NHS Plan*. London: The Stationery Office.

Department of Health (2000b) *National Service Framework for Coronary Heart Disease*. London: The Stationery Office.

Department of Health (2000c) *The National Cancer Plan*. London: The Stationery Office.

Department of Health (2001a) *Health and Social Care Act*. London: The Stationery Office.

Department of Health (2001b) *Primary Care General Practice and the NHS Plan*. London: The Stationery Office.

Department of Health (2001c) *Health Visitor Practice Resource Pack*. London: The Stationery Office.

Department of Health (2001d) *School Nurse Practice Resource Pack*. London: The Stationery Office.

Department of Health (2001e) *National Service Framework for Older People*. London: The Stationery Office.

Department of Health (2001f) *National Service Framework for Diabetes*. London: The Stationery Office.

Department of Health (2002a) *Liberating the Talents*. London: The Stationery Office.

Department of Health (2002b) *The Single Assessment Process for Older People*. London: The Stationery Office.

Department of Health (2002c) *Improvement, Expansion and Reform: The Next Three Years Priorities and Planning Framework 2003–06*. Available on line: www.Department of Health.gov.uk/planning2003-2006/index.htm

Department of Health (2003) *Supplementary Prescribing by Nurses and Pharmacists within the NHS in England: A Guide for Implementation*. London: DOH.

Department of Health and Social Services (1986) *Neighbourhood Nursing: A Focus for Care*. (Cumberlege Report). London: HMSO.

Goleman, D. (1998) *Working with Emotional Intelligence*. London: Bloomsbury.

Hannagan, T. (2000) *Management: Concepts and Practices*. London: Prentice Hall.

Hayes, D. (2000) The case against NHS Direct. *Doctor* (April): 36–9.

Hill, M.H. (2002) Transformational leadership in nursing education. *Nurse Educator*, 27(4): 162–4.

Human Rights Act (1998). London: The Stationery Office.

Johns, C. (1995) Framing learning through reflection within Carper's fundamental ways of knowing in nursing. *Journal of Advanced Nursing*, 22(2): 226–34.

McIntosh, J. (1996) The question of knowledge in district nursing. *International Journal of Nursing Studies*, 33(3): 316–24.

Medicinal Products: Prescription by Nurses Act (1992). London: HMSO.

Mental Health Act (1983). London: HMSO.

Nurses, Midwives and Health Visitors Act (1979). London: HMSO.

Nursing and Midwifery Council (2002) *Code of Professional Conduct.* London: NMC.

O'Cathain, A., Munro, J.F., Nicholl, J.P. and Knowles, E. (2000) How helpful is NHS Direct? A postal survey of callers. *British Medical Journal,* 320: 1035.

Ovretveit, J. (1997) How to describe interprofessional working. In J. Ovretveit, P. Mathias and T. Thompson (eds), *Interprofessional Working for Health and Social Care.* London: Macmillan.

Parsons, T. (1951) *The Social System.* London: Free Press.

Richards, D.A. and Tawfik, J. (2000) Introducing telephone triage into primary care nursing. *Nursing Standard,* 15(10): 42–5.

Robinson, J. and Elkan, R. (1996) *Health Needs Assessment: Theory and Practice.* Edinburgh: Churchill Livingstone.

Sadler, M. (2002) NHS Direct audited. Letter. *British Medical Journal,* 325: 164, 124.

Schon, D. (1991) *The Reflective Practitioner: How Professionals Think in Action.* Aldershot: Avebury.

Scottish Executive Health Department (2000) *Our National Health: A Plan for Change.* Edinbugh: The Stationery Office.

Scottish Executive Health Department (2001) *Nursing for Health: A Review of the Contribution of Nurses, Midwives and Health Visitors to Improving the Public's Health in Scotland.* Edinburgh: The Stationery Office.

Southard, D., Certo, C. and Comass, P. (1994) Core competencies for cardiac rehabilitation professionals. *Journal of Cardiopulmonary Rehabilitation,* 14: 87–92.

UK Central Council for Nursing, Midwifery and Health Visiting (1994) *The Future of Professional Practice: Standards for Community Specialist Practice.* London: UKCC.

Vanclay, L. (1998) Teamworking in primary care. *Nursing Standard,* 12(20): 37–8.

Worth, A. (1996) Identifying need for district nursing: towards a more proactive approach by practitioners. *NT Research,* 1(4): 260–9.

9

Nursing for public health

Sue Rouse, Sandra Baulcomb and Sandra Burley

Learning outcomes

- Evaluate the historical development of public health and the legacy for modern public health practice.
- Explain the origins of modern public health priorities and the determinants of health.
- Discuss the relevance of determinants of health to nursing practice.
- Identify the skills required for the improvement of public health and the contribution to be made by community nurses.

INTRODUCTION

Public health may by a relatively new topic for many nurses working in the community for the first time. This chapter seeks to develop the reader's understanding of the concept of public health and explores the actual and potential role for nurses in contributing to the public health agenda. It begins by defining public health and the evolution of public health care provision over the past hundred years. The reason for the current renewed emphasis on public health work is then considered by examination of some of the key policy developments, both international and national, over the past few decades. It is acknowledged that the NHS must have a role in caring for health as well as responding to ill health. The multi-disciplinary/multi-agency contribution to be made to the improvement of the health of the population is then explored with particular emphasis on the necessary and valuable role for nurses, especially community nurses. This is followed by some more detailed consideration of specific ways in which nurses can and should be using their skills and knowledge to contribute to the public health agenda with some ideas about how these activities can be incorporated into day-to-day practice.

WHAT IS PUBLIC HEALTH?

Exercise

For this exercise you will need access to several different newspapers all published on the same day. For example, a broadsheet (Times, Telegraph, Guardian); a 'blue top' tabloid (Daily Mail, Daily Express); a 'red top' tabloid (Mirror, Sun, Daily Star) and a local evening newspaper. *These may be accessed on the Internet or available in libraries.*

Look for reports in the newspapers of the same public health-related story – for example, the latest data on the prevalence of AIDS, or how asylum seekers are being processed and integrated into communities.

Read these reports, compare and contrast the way
the reports are written. What type of language is
used? Is blame apportioned to individuals or
collectively to institutions such as education, the
health service or the welfare state? Can you discern
a different approach or attitude towards the
problem? If so why do you think this is the case?
Can this be explained in relation to the way issues
on public heath are transmitted to the population
at large. What role can nurses play in ensuring the
population at large are well informed about public
health issues?

The term 'public health' has come to be used in two
separate but closely related ways. The first, refers to
the general state of health or wellbeing of the
population at large or the 'public'. The second is
used to describe those measures designed to care
for, maintain and promote such 'health' (Baggott
2000).

The meaning of the term has, however, changed
with time. As pointed out by Ashton and Seymour
(1988), both the general state of health of the
public and those measures designed to care for it
have evolved in line with the current state of
technological advancement and knowledge. Some
understanding of the historical context of 'public
health' may help to illustrate the modern usage of
the term.

During the 17th century, following the
population changes after the Industrial Revolution,
overcrowded and inadequate urban living
conditions led to the flourishing of infectious
diseases. Early attempts to combat this, through
improvements in housing, sanitation and education
about the importance of hygiene and clean food and
water, constituted the earliest organised public
health movement and included the appointment of
the first medical officers of health in Britain.
Following the discovery of germ theory and the
early availability of immunisation techniques during
the late 19th century, measures designed to improve
the health of the population shifted towards the
more personal preventive services. These services
included contraception, immunisation and clinic
services, and the health of the population became
less dominated by the ravages of infectious and
contagious disease.

From 1930 onwards, the discovery of insulin and
sulphonamides rendered a range of diseases more
susceptible to medical treatment and the
dominance of a curative approach to health care
became the reality. During this phase, the concept
of a population approach to public health measures
largely receded in favour of services focused on the
health needs of the individual.

Eventually, during the 1970s, it became apparent
that the purely therapeutic approach offered by
publicly funded medical interventions was both
insufficient and unsustainable in terms of cost and
effectiveness. There was a growing recognition that
a large proportion of modern disease was the result
of lifestyle changes and factors that could be
considered preventable prompted by a Canadian
report on the health of the population of Canada
(LaLonde 1974).

The current phase of public health activity has
been coined 'The New Public Health' and is
described as a phase which returns to the
consideration of environmental issues and
population health alongside those personal
preventive and therapeutic services which are now
well established (Ashton and Seymour 1988).
There is acknowledgement of the importance of the
social environment, policy and inequality as
determinants of the public's health experiences.

DEVELOPMENT OF THE PUBLIC HEALTH MOVEMENT

Table 9.1 shows the development of the public
health movement. Over the last 150 years four
distinct phases have emerged, reflecting changes in
society and developing knowledge and innovation
in health care. Tuberculosis (TB) has been chosen to
illustrate the change in emphasis over these phases.

Within the modern NHS, there is a recognition of
the important role of primary care and community
services in the prevention and promotion of health
as well as the treatment of disease (DOH 1997).
There is also some recognition of the limitations of
medicine alone in the provision of health care.
Medicine has traditionally focused on diseases and
their treatment using a physiological knowledge
base to underpin its practice. Nursing, on the other
hand, has tended to take a more holistic approach

Table 9.1

Era	Period	Characterised by:	Health gains achieved by:
Public health movement. Environmental change.	To: 1870s	Migration from countryside into towns. Poverty, overcrowding, poor sanitation. Infectious diseases such as TB predominate.	Improvements in housing, sanitation and the provision of safe clean water and food supplies help guard against the spread of TB.
Germ theory of disease. Individualistic approach.	To: 1930s	Emphasis now on personal preventive medical services. Immunisation, family planning.	Increased involvement of the state through provision of hospital and clinic services leads to improved individual health status and protection against TB.
Therapeutic era.	To: 1970s	Rising use of drugs and therapeutic interventions.	Move away from public health to hospital services and teaching hospitals. Sulphonamides used to treat TB.
New public health era.	To: present day	Escalating cost of health care. Technological innovation. Increasing demand for health care. Demographic changes, increase in elderly population.	Re-emphasis on environmental and personal preventive services alongside therapeutic intervention. Prevention of TB through immunisation and healthy public policy becomes the new focus.

to the care of individuals, incorporating broader definitions of health into its approaches to assessment and care planning.

The publication of the Acheson Report on health inequalities (1998) has prompted a new investigation into the determinants of ill health among the population at large. There is a renewed acknowledgement of the impact of factors such as employment, education, and the availability and accessibility of public services on the health experiences of both individuals and whole populations. The understanding of health in its wider form, beyond the presence or absence of disease and including social, emotional and spiritual factors is now more apparent. The impact of crime, substance misuse, homelessness, ethnicity and changing family patterns either directly or indirectly on the health experiences of the population, is acknowledged. Nurses, especially community-based nurses, are seen as having an important contribution to make to the care and improvement of the public's health. This can be achieved through both the direct provision of care and through collaboration with others and the influencing of policies that affect health both locally and nationally.

WHY PUBLIC HEALTH?

As indicated above, the limitations of a purely therapeutic approach to addressing modern health problems has long been acknowledged. International, national and local policies have recognised the need to combine programmes of ill-health prevention, health protection and health promotion alongside curative measures within health care provision (WHO 1981, 1998; DOH 1999a).

The World Health Organisation has been influential in the development of world policy. The role of primary health care services and the need for close co-operation between health care providers and other sectors, both statutory and voluntary, in the pursuit of improved public health is central to the objectives of their *Global Strategy for Health for All by the Year 2000* (WHO 1981). The targets were revised in 1998 in order to become applicable to Europe in the 21st century (WHO Regional Office for Europe 1998).

The publication of *The New NHS: Modern, Dependable* (DOH 1997) heralded the latest approach to improve health service provision in Britain. Building upon the recommendations of the Acheson Report (1998), along with subsequent guidance (DOH 2000), it emphasises the need for locally focused public health provision, proper consultation with service users, and modernisation of existing services to meet new demands.

Within nursing itself, a further overhaul of the profession and its approach to education outlined within *Making a Difference* (DOH 1999b) acknowledges the need for nurses to be highly educated, flexible and multi-skilled in order to meet the demands of modern health care. More recently, the government publication of *Liberating the Talents* (DOH 2002) has emphasised the need for creative approaches to co-operative and collaborative service provision, acknowledging the central role that specialist and generalist community nurses will have in the improvement of population health.

It would seem that escalating costs and ever-improving and technological advances within secondary care, may lead to limitations in the need for ever larger numbers of people accessing curative interventions. This represents a shift in favour of a broader and less costly population approach to the promotion and maintenance of better health. This becomes especially pertinent in the face of demographic shifts in population profiles, with fewer younger and middle-aged people available to care for the growing number of their frail older and disabled compatriots (www.statistics.gov.uk). It seems

imperative that those factors identified as determinants of poor health experiences and outcomes should be addressed as soon and as effectively as possible. This clearly means a widespread and collaborative approach between many national and local policy makers and service providers.

It has been argued that the very technological advances and publicly funded services that characterise the modern NHS in Britain can be held responsible for the decline in the health of the public that we appear to be now experiencing (Illich 1977). The welfare state has been blamed for encouraging people to shrug off personal responsibility for health status in the expectation that the NHS, paid for through taxes, will meet their health care needs as and when required.

The requirement for health needs assessment to be carried out at a local level has been central to NHS policy since the introduction of the internal market within the NHS in 1991 (DOH 1990). This has meant that local NHS organisations have had to develop the resources and expertise to enable them to obtain and analyse local health data. It is necessary to consult with the public and carry out local research to determine those factors which, if addressed effectively, are likely to lead to the most significant health gains. Since the eradication of the internal market, this requirement has become incorporated into the remit of local primary care trusts. The desire is to foster the production of local health improvement plans and focus health spending on services most relevant to local population health needs, including appropriate public health measures (DOH 1999a). Within such policy is an opportunity for community nurses to contribute to the gathering and interpretation of local data that will influence local policy (DOH 1995). Community nurses are in close and regular contact with users of primary care services and their families. This provides access to a rich source of data and information on population health experiences, attitudes and priorities that should be influential in determining local policy.

WHO HAS A ROLE IN PUBLIC HEALTH?

Perhaps the most readily identified role in public health is that of the Director of Public Health and the team of public health doctors, nurses, statisticians and researchers who work within the public health departments of local primary care trusts. These people, along with the Health Protection Agency have a clear remit within public health identified by the titles of their departments/services. The contribution of the work of local authority environmental health departments on public health priorities such as food hygiene, pest control and pollution is also readily identifiable.

There is recognition that the health of the public is affected by every aspect of their lives and environments. Factors which adversely affect the health of populations include those such as crime, substance misuse, transport and education. There is, then, a role for a wide range of services and agencies in tackling the public health agenda. The list of agencies with a significant contribution to make is likely to include every local authority department, including the police, education, transport, housing and social services as well as the more immediately identifiable role of the environmental health department, as mentioned above. In addition, many of the voluntary organisations which exist in any community are likely to have a significant part to play in promoting the health of the local population. Examples would include Homestart, Age Concern, National Society for the Prevention of Cruelty to Children, to name only a selection. The promotion, protection, maintenance and restoration of the health of the local population is clearly a task which must involve a broad range of agencies with a variety of roles and a range of expertise.

Exercise

Consider the residents of your own street, town or village and/or your own group of friends or relatives. In terms of their casual conversations across shop counters or at the bus stop what are the factors that concern people most? List the sorts of topics you hear people talking about and consider which of them may impact upon their health and how.

Now, look at your list and decide which of these topics can be addressed by a health professional, or health services alone and which may need the expertise of another service provider.

What proportion of the factors you listed can be addressed using the expertise of health professionals? What does this tell you about the range of agencies which have a role in the tackling of public health issues?

At the level of local health services, co-ordinating the promotion, maintenance and improvement of the health of the population is the remit of the primary care trusts. This role clearly requires a set of skills which are different from but complementary to those required in the secondary care, curative services, sometimes most readily associated with medical and health service provision and provided by hospital-centred NHS trusts. Some knowledge of physical and mental health and the contributory factors for ill health and disease can be a clear advantage in some aspects of public health work, but the knowledge and expertise required goes beyond these specialist areas.

Essentially, public health work must involve a process of population health needs assessment, including analysis and processing of data in order to gain an understanding of the factors which contribute to both good and poor health. Public health work includes providing services or influencing service provision in such a way as to seek to eliminate adverse factors and to promote positive ones. As in all aspects of care and under the guidance of clinical governance (NHSME 1999; Swage 2000) these processes must be followed by the careful evaluation of outcomes in order to inform a cycle of improvement. This sequence of activities has much in common with the systematic approach to nursing care or 'the nursing process' taught to and used by nurses of every discipline. The major difference in using the model for public health purposes is that the skills and knowledge involved in the assessment, planning, implementation and evaluation of care must be applied to a population rather than an individual. The direct provision of nursing care may be replaced by the influencing or organisation of care/services at a more strategic level, often in collaboration with others. It is clear, however, that there is a correlation between the motivation (better health), skills (assessment, planning, implementation and evaluation) and knowledge base (factors which affect health) of nurses and those required for public health work. Nurses' therefore are perceived as having a significant role to play.

Exercise

Think about your role in assessment, planning, implementation and evaluation of care for an individual patient or client you have cared for in the past. What are the skills you needed to use at each of these stages of the nursing process? Now think about how you would go about assessing the collective health needs of the people living on a small local housing estate? What skills would you need to use?

Did either of your lists include the following skills?

Assessment	Planning
Communication	Communication
Record-keeping	Teaching
Listening	Negotiation
Data analysis	Application of
research	
Empathy	knowledge to
practice	

Implementation	Evaluation
Delegation	Data analysis
Record-keeping	Synthesis
Communication	
Clinical skills	
Liaison	
Referral	

Government policy has clearly indicated the need for nurses to become more involved in improving the health of the population and public health work. Relatively early policy documents made specific reference to the contribution that nurses could and should make in the field of public health. In the last decade national strategies for improving the nation's health set out a clear role for nurses, among others, in health promotion and prevention of ill health, through provision of education and support and influencing policy (NHSME 1993; DOH 1992, 1995, 1998, 2000, 2002).

It is clear that the health of the population and particularly the huge inequalities experienced by people from different backgrounds and even different geographical areas is determined by factors other than the provision and/or quality of medical or health services available (Acheson 1998). It is now evident that people from the lower socio-economic groups are more likely to suffer prematurely from heart disease than those from the higher socio-economic groups, for instance. It is equally apparent that the rates of morbidity and mortality are higher in the less affluent geographical areas of the country than the more affluent. Socio-economic variants, such as employment and housing, then, have an impact on life expectancy and general health status.

There have been concerted health education campaigns encouraging people to modify their lifestyles in order to guard against the early development of diseases such as coronary heart disease and stroke. Nurses, alongside health education/health promotion experts, are seen as being among those in the front line in terms of such health education. Subsequently, it has become clear that the very factors that characterise inequalities in health status also mitigate against the ability of people to make the desired lifestyle decisions. The focus of public health campaigns has thus moved towards 'making the healthier choices the easier choices' (DOH 1998). This requires changes in policy in the fields of environment, the economy, education and transport, among others in order for such a goal to be achieved. Nurse training stresses the importance of effective communication skills (NMC 2002a), with the users of their services, each other and, the multi-disciplinary and multi-agency team members who contribute to any health care plan. Nurses, therefore, already have in place networks of communication that can be strengthened and utilised at all levels in order to enhance a multi-agency approach to the improvement of health experiences- both for individuals and for communities.

Planning for public health needs access to knowledge about the health status of the local population, factors that contribute to this, and evaluation of those services which are already in existence to help improve people's health. Nurses working in the community in primary care settings have access to people within their own living environment. Such contact allows nurses access to the 'soft' data which is required for a comprehensive assessment of local health needs. This information cannot be gathered from epidemiological studies alone but must be enhanced by access to information obtained directly from those people at risk of poor health experiences. There is, therefore, a significant influence which community nurses can exert upon local policy making by collating and providing such essential data to inform local health improvement plans.

The combination of medical and nursing expertise and data collection can thus provide a complementary and effective way of working towards a local public health strategy. Efffective working relationships with the local authority and voluntary organisations can ensure the success of schemes such as 'Healthy Schools' projects (www.wiredforhealth.gov.uk), Sure Start (www.surestart.gov.uk), Healthy Cities (Davies and Kelly 1992), and others.

The real expertise in terms of understanding and contributing to their own health outcomes comes from the public itself. Recent developments in both policy and practice acknowledge the value of community development initiatives as a way forward in fostering the health of communities. Professionals take on the role of facilitators in terms of engaging representatives of local communities in both determining their own health priorities and the local response. The result can take the form of direct service development or lobbying of policy makers to fund and provide services as determined by the local population. There are some good examples of success in terms of community development which take true cognisance of the expertise of local people in understanding and taking responsibility for responding to their own health needs; see Valois (2003) and Carter and El-Hassan (2003).

HOW CAN NURSES CONTRIBUTE TO PUBLIC HEALTH OUTCOMES?

Working in partnership with patients and clients and encouraging them to take responsibility for decision-making about their own health can lead to more effective 'bottom-up' solutions to experienced/anticipated health problems. Through negotiating with clients nurses can achieve better outcomes than can be gained through a more prescriptive approach

to the provision of health care. For example the Medicines Partnership have done considerable work to encourage concordance in connection with the prescription of medicines as an aid to improving outcomes (Carter and Taylor 2003). This can be further extended beyond work with individuals to working with groups and communities in a community development way so that members of the community themselves become engaged in and/or responsible for identifying their own health needs and designing/commissioning their own interventions to meet those needs. This 'bottom–up' way of working reduces the wastage of resources on the development of expensive but unsuitable resources which are subsequently unused or poorly used by the people for whom they are intended. This has been a feature of health care provision for many years and was remarked upon by Tudor Hart (1972), who observed that services were often accessed most by those who were likely to benefit least and remained inaccessible to those who might most benefit and for whom they may have been designed. Such a phenomenon has contributed to the perpetuation of inequalities of health as highlighted by Acheson (1998).

Example

When the issue of high rates of teenage pregnancy first came to the fore, there was a flurry of developments around specialist contraception services in order to inform, educate and supply young people with access to better methods of contraception and thus seek to avoid unwanted pregnancies. However, comprehensive holistic assessment and further research led to the realisation that some young people actually planned their early pregnancies and saw parenthood as a way of gaining recognition by wider society in terms of access to suitable housing and benefits and the ability to perform a useful social role with important and fulfilling relationships. This, in turn has led to some innovative schemes which seek to explore issues about relationships, parenthood and self-esteem among young people and *thus address some of the broader social factors associated with teenage parenthood.*

Nurses can also be instrumental in ensuring the optimum use of local resources. By being aware of and working alongside other agencies, both statutory and voluntary, community nurses can refer patients/clients to receive the range of services which will best meet their identified health needs and can also influence the way in which local services develop. For example, community nurses can work alongside agencies such as Age Concern to develop Carer Support services and ensure that people are appropriately referred and well-supported in their important caring roles.

Another way in which nurses' regular and unique contact with people at home can contribute to policy making is in helping to ensure appropriate consumer involvement in decision making. There has been a growing trend in public policy (DOH 1997, 2000) to involve users of services directly in the decision making relating to local service provision. Nurses can play a significant role in encouraging service users to become involved in consultation exercises or by advocating for those unwilling to become directly involved.

The significant contribution to be made in the field of public health by nurses has recently been recognised in the development of nurse consultant posts in public health. Increasing numbers of PCT public health departments now have one or more specialist public health nurses within the team. These specialist senior and experienced nurses work alongside their medical and other colleagues to ensure that nursing data and expertise is both developed and utilised in this field. The further development of the curriculum for public health nurses (NMC 2002b) to re-establish the principles of health visiting or public health nursing as the basis for teaching and training is likely to reinforce the role to be played by nurses in supporting public health developments for many years to come.

WHERE AND WHEN CAN NURSING FOR PUBLIC HEALTH OCCUR?

All nursing interventions are aimed at contributing to health improvements, either for individuals or groups. Activities that range from the treatment of leg ulcers to the education and reassurance of young teenage parents, all have the aim of improving

health in its widest sense. In this way, community nurses have a daily contribution to make in improving the public's health.

They may use their contact with individuals and families in their own homes to educate people about those factors which may be affecting their health and ways of dealing with them. This may be carried out directly through behaviour change or indirectly through referral to available services. Additionally this information can be used to inform local health planning.

Analysis and interpretation of local health data may indicate the need for community nursing services themselves to be organised and delivered differently in order to make a greater impact upon the health of the population (DOH 2002). For example, district nurses may be able to carry out an assessment of a client's home environment and medication status in order to put in place measures designed to reduce the incidence of falls amongst older people. This could take place at the same time as responding to an established health need such as wound care or administration of medicines. Access to appropriate health care services may be improved by taking services to people who are likely to benefit most from them rather than expecting them to visit a surgery or clinic. For example, services for older people may be provided in a local day centre or residential establishment and services for children and families could be provided from a nursery or play group premises. In this way, services may be rendered less threatening and more relevant to the everyday lives of the individuals for whose benefit they are intended.

Providing valuable data to contribute to the local health needs assessment process and thus to influence service development and policy making can become a routine part of daily practice. This function could be greatly enhanced through the use of information technology systems designed for the purpose of collecting and collating valuable health data.

Exercise

Revisit the questions raised in the first exercise. On reflection in the light of your reading have your views changed?

Public health can be addressed through the daily nursing practice of all community nurses, once they are aware of the contribution they can make and are able to adjust their practice to accommodate this important social function.

FURTHER READING

Department of Health (2001) *On the State of the Public Health. The Annual Report of the Chief Medical Office of the Department of Health.* London: DOH.

Plews, C., Billingham, K. and Rowe, A. (2000) Public health nursing; barriers and opportunities. *Health and Social Care in the Community,* 8(2): 138–46.

Websites

The following websites are useful sources of up-to-date information on public health and associated nursing issues.

Department of Health
www.doh.gov.uk/public.htm
Health Development Agency
www.hda-online.org.uk
Health Protection Agency
www.hpa.org.uk
National Healthy School Standard
www.wiredforhealth.gov.uk
Nursing and Midwifery Council
www.nmc-uk.org
Public Health Laboratory Service
www.phls.org.uk
Surestart
www.surestart.gov.uk
World Health Organisation
www.whodk/informationsources

REFERENCES

Acheson, D. (1998) *Report of the Independent Inquiry into Inequalities in Health* (Acheson Report). London: Stationery Office.

Ashton, J. and Seymour, H. (1988) *The New Public Health.* Milton Keynes: Open University.

Baggott, R. (2000) *Public Health: Policy and Politics.* Basingstoke: Macmillan.

Carter, M. and El-Hassan, A.A. (2003) *Between NASS and a Hard Place: Refugee Housing and Community Development on Yorkshire and Humberside. A Feasibility Study.* London: Housing Associations' Charitable Trust.

Carter, S. and Taylor, D. (2003) *A Question of Choice: Compliance in Medicine Taking.* London: Medicines Partnership.

Davies, J. and Kelly, M. (eds) (1992) *Healthy Cities: Policy and Practice.* London: Routledge.

Department of Health (1990) *NHS and Community Care Act.* London: HMSO.

Department of Health (1992) *Health of the Nation: A Strategy for Health in England* (Cmnd 1986). London: HMSO.

Department of Health, Standing Nursing and Midwifery Advisory Committee (1995) *Making it Happen: Public Health: The Contribution , Role and Development of Nurses, Midwives and Health Visitors.* London: HMSO.

Department of Health (1997) *The New NHS: Modern, Dependable* (Cmnd 3807). London: The Stationery Office.

Department of Health (1998) *Our Healthier Nation.* London: HMSO.

Department of Health (1999a) *Saving Lives: Our Healthier Nation.* London: The Stationery Office.

Department of Health (1999b) *Making a Difference: Strengthening the Nursing, Midwifery and Health Visiting Contribution to Health and Healthcare.* London: The Stationery Office.

Department of Health (2000) *The NHS Plan.* London: The Stationery Office.

Department of Health (2002) *Liberating the Talents.* London: The Stationery Office.

Department of Health and Social Security (1976) *Prevention and Health: Everybody's Business.* London: HMSO.

Illich, I. (1977) *Limits to Medicine. Medical Nemesis: The Expropriation of Health.* London: Pelican.

LaLonde, M. (1974) *A New Perspective on the Health of Canadians.* Ottawa: Government of Canada.

NHS Management Executive (1993) *New World, New Opportunities: Nursing in Primary Health Care.* London: HMSO.

NHS Management Executive (1993) *A Vision for the Future.* London: HMSO.

NHS Management Executive (1999) *A First Class Service: Quality in the New NHS.* London: HMSO.

Nursing and Midwifery Council (2002a) *Requirements for Pre-registration Health Visitor Programmes.* London: NMC.

Nursing and Midwifery Council (2002b) *Requirements for Pre-registration Nurse Programmes.* London: NMC.

Swage, T. (2000) *Clinical Governance in Health Care Practice.* Oxford, Butterworth–Heinemann.

Tudor Hart, J. (1972) The inverse care law. *Lancet*: 405–12.

Valois, N. (2003) Extend yourself. *Community Care*, 15 May: 32–5.

World Health Organisation (1981) *Global Strategy for Health for All by the Year 2000.* Geneva: WHO.

World Health Organisation Regional Office for Europe (1998) *Health 21: The Health for All Policy Framework for the Twenty-first Century.* Copenhagen: WHO.

www.statistics.gov.uk

www.surestart.gov.uk

www.wiredforhealth.gov.uk

10

Developing health promotion practice

Karen Melling, Judy Gleeson and Karen Hunter

Learning outcomes

- Discuss definitions and underlying principles of health promotion.
- Explore a range of core competencies of health promotion.
- Review own levels of competence in health promotion and identify potential strategies for their development.
- Identify opportunities for applying the competencies into your current practice.

INTRODUCTION

It is acknowledged that you will have considered aspects of health promotion theory and practice within your pre-registration training, however this chapter will explore a number of different aspects of the current debate related to health promotion, following on from a brief review of the concept of health.

Health promotion is part of a wider public health agenda, which is discussed in detail in Chapter 9. Here we will be focusing on the approaches and competencies you will need to support the delivery of effective health promotion interventions as one strand of public health development. It is hoped this will enable you to gain a better understanding of what health promotion is about, how it is 'done' and what competencies you need to be able to integrate health promotion into your on-going practice within the community.

It is beyond the scope of this chapter to cover the theory of health promotion in detail. Therefore we have included a range of further reading, which you may wish to pursue to expand your understanding in this area and further contextualise your practice.

WHAT IS HEALTH?

Any attempt to define health promotion fundamentally needs to give some consideration to the question, 'What is health?' The concept of 'health' has long been a contested one, ranging from Mansfield's view of health as personal fulfilment – 'by health I mean the power to live a full, adult, living, breathing life in close contact with what I love … I want to be all that I am capable of becoming' (Mansfield 1977: p. 278) – through to a more specific medical model view which sees health predominantly as the absence of disease.

This, in the past, has been a dominant paradigm adopted by many health care professionals, although there has been a shift towards the adoption of a more holistic definition of health such as that of the World Health Organisation:

> [Health is] the extent to which an individual or group is able, on the one hand, to realise aspirations and satisfy needs; and, on the other hand, to change or cope with the environment. Health is, therefore, seen as a resource for everyday life, not an object of living; it is a

positive concept emphasising social and personal resources as well as physical capacities.

(WHO 1984)

The scope of this chapter does not allow for an in-depth consideration of this issue. For a wider debate on the contested concept of health further reading is suggested at the end of this chapter, including Seedhouse (1997) and Naidoo and Wills (2000).

> ### Exercise
>
> What does 'being healthy' mean to you?

There are no right or wrong answers to this question; your thoughts may have covered aspects of physical, mental, spiritual, social and sexual health and will have been influenced by your personal life experiences. It is important to recognise these influences and also how other people, both professionals and lay people, may well experience different sets of influences which will colour their perceptions of this concept of 'being healthy'.

WHAT IS HEALTH PROMOTION?

There are numerous definitions of health promotion in the literature, reflecting both the breadth of health promotion practice and also the issues around the contested concept of 'health'. It may well depend on your preferred definition of health as to which of the definitions of health promotion you are most comfortable with.

Here are two examples of definitions of health promotion for you to consider:

> Health promotion is the process of enabling people to increase control over, and to improve, their health.
>
> (WHO 1984)

> Health promotion comprises the efforts to enhance positive health and prevent ill-health, through the overlapping spheres of health education, prevention and health protection. Empowerment is a cardinal principle of health promotion.
>
> (Downie *et al.* 1996)

Both definitions indicate that health promotion is something which is 'done' to achieve a particular goal or outcome, here defined in terms such as 'improving health, 'enhancing positive health' and 'preventing ill health'.

> ### Exercise
>
> Why do health professionals and others undertake health promotion activities? Take a moment to consider, from your perspective, what the goals of health promotion are.

In considering the goals of health promotion you may have come up with a number of different reasons in your list, such as:

* to secure better health for people as individuals or as a community or wider population
* to reduce inequalities in health between groups in the population
* to reduce the incidence of preventable disease such as coronary heart disease or cancer
* to increase life expectancy within the population;
* to enhance someone's quality of life
* to meet National Service Framework targets.

All of these broad goals would be seen as valid reasons for undertaking some health promotion activity and, indeed, all of them are embedded in the current political agenda for health, as identified in documents such as *Saving Lives: Our Healthier Nation* (DOH 1999), *The NHS Plan* (DOH 2000) and the various *National Service Frameworks* (DOH 1999, 2000, 2001). (These policies are discussed further in Chapter 9.)

This chapter is written from the perspective that health promotion is an umbrella term which embraces activities in one, some or all of the following areas: health education programmes, preventive health services, community-based work, organisational development, economic and regulatory activities, environmental health measures and healthy public policies (as identified by Ewles and Simnett 2003).

Within this diverse collection of activities the breadth, level and depth of any activity is very wide-ranging – from an individual community staff nurse engaged in a one-to-one discussion with a patient, giving advice on healthy eating, to a nurse influencing health promotion issues at policy level: for example, a nurse member of the professional executive committee of a primary care trust developing healthy eating strategies for children and young people as part of the local development plan.

In considering the opportunities for incorporating health promotion into your practice it is important to bear in mind the principles on which health promotion should be grounded. These were outlined by the WHO in 1984 as follows:

- Health promotion involves the population as a whole in the context of their everyday life, rather than focusing on people at risk of contracting specific diseases.
- Health promotion is directed towards action on the causes or determinants of health.
- Health promotion combines diverse, but complementary, methods or approaches.
- Health promotion aims particularly at effective and concrete public participation.
- While health promotion is basically an activity in the health and social fields, and not a medical service, health professionals – particularly in primary care – have an important role in nurturing and enabling health promotion.

The practice of health promotion will require you to look critically at your own values and attitudes in relation to health behaviours, both of your own and your clients. As in nursing practice there is a need to be non-judgemental in your approach, working with individuals and communities to achieve 'health' as they determine it, not as you would impose upon them. As has been identified in the Tannahill's definition of health promotion, quoted above, a fundamental element is that of empowering individuals and communities to identify their own health needs and set their own agenda for health gain. This process will require an ability to work with clients rather than directing them in a particular direction.

It is important to take into account influences such as culture, religion, gender, sexual orientation, disability, socio-economic grouping and how they impact on the individual's value system that may, in turn, impinge on their choices in relation to health behaviour.

In summary, you need to adopt an appropriate approach and/or select a suitable activity, that is inclusive of the individual or client group, taking account of the influences impinging on health for that individual or community.

As is indicated in the WHO principles of health promotion, it is important to recognise and acknowledge that no health promotion activity is the exclusive responsibility of any one professional group or discipline; working with others in partnership and collaboration is an important approach to adopt. However, nurses working in the community often have a role in facilitating and/or participating in many health-promoting activities which, if applied appropriately, will work towards achieving positive health outcomes for individual patients or clients and within local communities.

WHAT COMPETENCIES DO YOU NEED FOR EFFECTIVE HEALTH PROMOTION?

The breadth of health promotion requires diverse competencies, related to the areas of activity in which you are engaged. Competencies include components of knowledge, skills and attitude. This chapter will now go on to explore ways in which your existing competencies can be applied and developed further in relation to health promotion practice.

Many nurses working in the community have long recognised the importance of health promotion within their role. However, when questioned they may say that they do not 'do health promotion'. Indeed, much health promotion takes place whilst other procedures or interventions are being carried out: it is integral to the role and not seen as something different or extra. However, it is perhaps worth reflecting on what within your work could be classified as 'health promotion'. Sometimes the challenge is undertaking health promotion activities alongside other competing demands.

Exercise

Consider for a moment a client you have cared for recently and bring to mind any health-promoting or health-enhancing activities you may have undertaken. Reflect on which competencies you have used.

Within the field of health promotion Ewles and Simnett (2003) have identified a number of core competencies that can be built on and developed as you have the opportunity and gain experience in integrating health promotion into your practice. Although these have been identified as separate competencies they are closely interrelated and often elements from each area of competence will be drawn upon within a specific health promotion activity or initiative.

- managing, planning and evaluating
- educating
- communicating
- facilitating and networking
- marketing and publicity
- influencing policy and practice.

It is important to recognise that these competencies are not exclusive to health promotion; indeed, it is acknowledged that you will have developed many of them already through initial nurse education programmes, through life experiences and, subsequently, in practice. However, you may wish to consider how these competencies relate to health promotion practice within the community setting. In order to deliver the health promotion agenda, you are likely to draw on, and develop further, skills and competence in some or all of these areas.

The following section will expand on each of the areas of competence, outlining some of the essential elements and providing examples of how the competencies might be utilised in practice.

Managing, planning and evaluation

In any health promotion activity, it is important to be clear about what you are trying to achieve and how you are going to go about it. This requires you to plan and manage your activity systematically, setting realistic and clear aims and objectives, selecting appropriate methods of delivery and also, at an early stage, identifying your evaluation tools. Consideration also needs to be given to the resources you have available, including time, money, personnel and access to equipment and facilities. In undertaking this you should be able to develop a

project plan that will incorporate a realistic timeframe for delivery.

Such planning may be done by an individual, a small working group or team of staff, perhaps involving people from other disciplines or other agencies who also have a role in promoting the health of the local population. This 'working together' or working in partnership encourages a sharing of ideas and resources and may expand the potential opportunities within the activity being planned. It is important to identify who will 'lead' the project or activity. Steering a boat without a rudder is a recipe for disaster! Also remember to keep notes of all decisions and actions to be taken, including who is responsible for each part of the project so that everyone is clear about what is expected of them. For more detail on the planning process in health promotion see Ewles and Simnett (2003) and Naidoo and Wills (2000).

Evaluation is an important part of any health promotion activity: it allows you to measure your success, learn from your experiences and plan for the future. This need not be a complex or onerous task but it is an important one. If possible share your potential evaluation methods with someone, such as a senior colleague, health promotion specialist, line manager. There are numerous tools and guides to evaluation which may be helpful to you, for example see Peberdy (cited in Katz *et al.* 2000).

Example

A staff nurse in the health visiting team may be able to support the specialist practitioner in developing materials for display at the market health stall as part of a health fair promoting healthy eating. The role would encompass elements of forward planning, implementation and evaluation, working alongside other team members.

Educating

Education is a key tool in promoting health, and health promoters will be using this competency in a variety of ways and settings, from the formal teaching of large groups in schools to informal input on a one-to-one basis in a clinic or nursing home. In undertaking any educating role it is important to plan your input, make sure you are up-to-date with the knowledge base, think about the most appropriate style of delivery, such as a didactic approach, where you have limited time and a large group, to a more Socratic approach, with a small group in which interaction can be encouraged. Again, the measuring of success of your delivery is an important aspect of this intervention. Fundamental to this area of competence is effective communication.

Example

A school nurse specialist may need support in developing a hand-washing programme for primary school children. Here the E- or D-grade nurse may work with the school children to create place mats with pictures depicting good hand-washing practices.

Communicating

This area of competence will not be new to you. Communication is a fundamental skill for all health professionals and one which is used constantly. It is also fundamental to health promotion practice. We can communicate with our clients in many different ways and it is important to select the most appropriate for the situation. How we communicate with people, when we communicate with people and what we communicate to people are all important aspects to consider.

Exercise

How many ways of communicating health messages can you think of?

Health promoting messages can be delivered through many media, but for maximum effectiveness, it is important to match up the person, the message and the method of communication. Communicating health messages can take many forms, including one-to-one advice from a health professional, group teaching in schools by school nurses, posters and leaflets, health fairs, videos, NHS Direct, through the internet, telephone helplines, newspapers and magazines, television and radio.

Examples

The use of the *Smokebuster* magazine/comic to encourage young people to quit smoking.

An E-grade nurse working in the community with the district nursing team arranging for a local older peoples' drama group to perform a play about reducing accidents in the home to clients attending the local Age Concern luncheon club and day centre.

Facilitating and networking

It is important to recognise how other people can help you in your health promoting role and how you can help others. Sharing ideas, skills and knowledge is all part of this, particularly when working with local communities and groups and other organisations. Getting to know what is happening locally and who is involved is an important and useful process.

Working together with others on projects can help to enhance the effectiveness of the activity and helps to share the workload. This is an important aspect to consider when you want to incorporate health promotion work into an already busy schedule.

Examples

A community mental health nurse working with carers to establish a local carers' self-help/support group.

Attending the annual general meeting of a local support group to find out more about what is happening and who is involved.

Marketing and publicity

Raising awareness of your health promotion activities can be important to support you in sharing good practice, widening participation in the activities and providing further opportunities for promoting the health messages. This can be done in a variety of ways from an informal approach using a poster display in the local surgery through to seeking support from the local press for a major health event in the town. There will be people in your local primary care trust with particular skills in liaising with the press who can help you with developing publicity materials. It may be necessary to gain approval for any press releases you might want to make related to particular projects in which you are involved.

Example

An occupational health nurse developing and displaying publicity material on the flu vaccination campaign in their local workplace.

Influencing policy and practice

You may feel that your opportunities in this area are limited. However, participating in audits, recording activities undertaken to identify trends in local populations, being involved in pilot projects, sharing good practice and fully participating in local staff meetings all provide the potential to influence policy and practice at a local level.

A focus on evidence-based practice is important, ensuring you and your work colleagues are delivering a quality-based service to the local population. (See Chapter 2 for a discussion of clinical governance.)

Taking a pro-active approach to your health promotion activities can provide opportunities to influence practice and can lead to greater satisfaction with your work. Why not find out if your trust offers a reward scheme for 'good ideas'; many do.

There are also opportunities you can take as an individual citizen, such as voting for your local council representatives or standing as a representative yourself, or participating in local consultation processes, such as the closure of a local health facility.

Example

Community staff nurses supporting the running and evaluation of a pilot scheme for a community-based leg ulcer clinic to influence future provision.

HOW DO YOU DEVELOP THESE COMPETENCIES?

Developing competence in health promotion practice often involves the enhancement of existing skills and knowledge, and incorporating them into new or different ways of working. It is about transferring skills across into a new domain or area of practice.

Exercise

Reflecting on the list of core competencies, in which areas do you feel you have existing 'transferable skills' and where is there room for development?

Using a tool such as a SLOT analysis might assist you in this task. A SLOT analysis encourages you to consider the task, focusing on the following areas: strengths, limitations, opportunities and threats.

Self-assessment of levels of competence is not always an easy task. You could be helped to do this through a variety of channels including, for example, preceptorship, clinical supervision, individual performance review or staff development review, reflective practice and feedback from colleagues and clients.

Levels of competence and consequent learning needs will vary from individual to individual, depending on previous experience and learning opportunities. You may have come into nursing following a career in marketing, in which case your competence in that area may well be high whereas your experience in educating others is very limited Or you may have just completed your nurse education, having come direct from school, and the opportunities to date for you to develop your competence in areas such as facilitating and networking have been limited, whereas your competence in communicating with individual clients is high. Or you may have undertaken a health studies degree, which included modules on health promotion, that has given you a substantial grounding in the area although this may focus more on the theory and knowledge base rather than the application in practice.

Whatever the circumstances for you as an individual, having assessed your competency levels it is possible to look for opportunities to enhance those competencies you identify as needing development. Again, how you achieve this will vary, depending on the area of competence, your personal and work circumstances and the level of support available to you through your workplace.

One effective way of developing competence is through experiential learning, by applying the skills in practice, with support as necessary in the first instance, and to reflect on the process and the outcome. This is perhaps best supported by a senior colleague or manager who is already experienced in the field and who can coach or mentor you through the learning process. This will obviously require you to be given the opportunity to incorporate some health promotion practice into your work programme and this may need to be facilitated with support from other colleagues. Another source of help and support could be through your local public health, health improvement or health promotion colleagues who should be able to offer specialist advice and guidance in the field to help you in applying the skills to practice and providing the appropriate evidence base to assist in directing your practice.

Another opportunity that will almost certainly offer new experiences and perspectives from which you can learn and develop is through participating in inter-agency projects or initiatives. As has been indicated previously, working in partnership with others is an important aspect of health promotion activity and one which should be taken up where feasible. It is potentially a new and challenging

experience for many staff, but one that can be rewarding and enriching, enabling you to expand your existing competence and develop others. Again, if this way of working is new to you it is suggested you undertake such activity with support and supervision from more experienced colleagues in the first instance, and also take the opportunity to reflect on the process and practice. Use of a reflective model, such as those of Gibbs (1988) or Johns (1996), may assist you in this task.

It may be that you have identified underpinning knowledge gaps, rather than specific skills gaps. If this is the case the means of meeting your learning needs will probably be different from those suggested previously. For example, you may benefit from undertaking some specific focused reading around the topic concerned, attending an update session on falls prevention for the elderly (if that is the area of knowledge deficit) or perhaps preparing a seminar paper for your colleagues on an area of work relevant to the team, such as reducing the problems of obesity among young people. Again the specialist public health and health improvement/promotion staff should be a good source of help and support.

Opportunities for learning and enhancing competency levels in health promotion will vary across the country and the suggestions made here are only examples. You will need to clarify your learning needs, make those needs known to your manager and then seek appropriate opportunities to meet those needs, based on the situation locally.

CONCLUSION

To meet the requirements of the current agenda for health improvement there is a need for staff in a wide range of roles and settings to adopt a proactive health promotion element in their work. We hope that this chapter has inspired you to feel confident in developing your competencies to enhance the health of your client group and that it has illustrated how health promotion can be something that is integrated into your everyday activity.

Engaging in health promotion can be many things for you as a practitioner: challenging, exciting, frustrating, rewarding, at times overwhelming, enjoyable, innovative, empowering, satisfying, time-consuming, skill-enhancing, self-actualising, stressful, but overall very worthwhile. Wherever and whenever health-promoting opportunities arise we urge you to participate actively.

FURTHER READING

Ewles, L. and Simnett, I. (2003) *Promoting Health: A Practical Guide (5th edn)*. Edinburgh: Baillière Tindall/RCN.

Katz, J., Peberdy, A. and Douglas, J. (eds) (2000) *Promoting Health: Knowledge and Practice (2nd edn)*. Basingstoke: Palgrave in association with the Open University.

Naidoo, J. and Wills, J. (2000) *Health Promotion: Foundation for Practice* Edinburgh: Baillière Tindall /RCN.

Seedhouse, D. (1997) *Health Promotion: Philosophy, Prejudice and Practice*. Chichester; John Wiley.

REFERENCES

Downie, R.S., Tannahill, C. and Tannahill A. (1996) *Health Promotion: Models and Values (2nd edn)*. Oxford: Oxford Medical Publications.

Department of Health (1999) *Saving Lives: Our Healthier Nation*. London: The Stationery Office.

Department of Health (1999) *Mental Health National Health Service Framework*. London: The Stationery Office.

Department of Health (2000) *The NHS Plan*. London: The Stationery Office.

Department of Health (2000) *Coronary Heart Disease National Health Service Framework*. London: The Stationery Office.

Department of Health (2001) *Older People National Health Service Framework*. London: The Stationery Office.

Ewles, L. and Simnett, I. (2003) *Promoting Health: A Practical Guide (5th edn)*. Edinburgh: Baillière Tindall/RCN.

Gibbs, G. (1988) *Learning by Doing: A Guide to Teaching and Learning Methods*. Oxford: Oxford Polytechnic.

Johns, C. (1996) Visualizing and realising caring in practice through guided reflection. *Journal of Advanced Nursing* 24: 1/35–43.

Katz, J., Peberdy, A. and Douglas, J. (eds) (2000) *Promoting Health: Knowledge and Practice*. Basingstoke: Palgrave in association with the Open University.

Naidoo, J. and Wills, J. (2000) *Health Promotion: Foundation for Practice*. Edinburgh: Baillière Tindall /RCN.

Seedhouse, D. (1997) *Health Promotion: Philosophy, Prejudice and Practice*. Chichester: John Wiley.

World Health Organisation (1984) *Health Promotion: A Discussion Document on the Concept and Principles*. Copenhagen: WHO Regional Office for Europe.

Index